Temporal Bone

Surgical Anatomy

A Colour Atlas of Temporal Bone Surgical Anatomy

R. T. Counter

Surgeon Lieutenant Commander
MB, BS, FRCS (Ed), DLO, Royal Navy

Wolfe Medical Publications Ltd

Published by Wolfe Medical Publications Ltd, 1980
Printed by Smeets-Weert, Holland
ISBN 0 7234 0749 5 Cased edition
ISBN 0 7234 1609 5 Paperback edition

For a full list of Wolfe Medical Atlases, plus forthcoming titles and details of our surgical, dental and veterinary Atlases, please write to Wolfe Publishing Ltd, 2-16 Torrington Place, London WC1E 7LT.

General Editor, Wolfe Medical Atlases:
G. Barry Carruthers, MD(Lond)

A CIP catalogue record for this book is available from the British Library.

Contents

Acknowledgements

This Atlas would not have become possible without the invaluable help of the Photographic and Radiographic Departments at the Royal Naval Hospital, Haslar, Portsmouth, Hampshire.

The author would like to thank the MOIC, RNH Haslar and the Medical Director General (Naval) for their assistance in making possible the production of this book, and Professor R. M. H. McMinn and Mr R. T. Hutchings, both of the Royal College of Surgeons of England, for permission to use pictures 2, 3, 5, 7, 11, 13, 15, 17 and 20 which are from "A Colour Atlas of Human Anatomy" (Wolfe Medical Publications Ltd).

Introduction

The aim of this atlas is to elucidate a fascinating but complicated subject—the petrous temporal bone. I hope it will be useful not only to those preparing for specialist examinations, but to anyone studying the dissection of the temporal bone area.

The temporal bone area is difficult to visualise in three dimensions from description alone. In the past it has been the practice to use heavily annotated line drawings, which become so stylised that the true appearance is lost. I have tried to overcome this drawback by the use of colour photography to show temporal bone dissections from a variety of angles and so build up a comprehensive picture of the anatomy.

The dissections are of dried temporal bones and every effort has been made to provide both views of the bones as seen at surgery and more unusual views to help understand the anatomy. A three dimensional understanding of the anatomy is probably more essential in this area than in most others, and I have tried to supply colour illustrations which encourage this type of understanding.

Modern radiology of the temporal bone, using standard views and polytomography has been included in each section, not only because it assists in learning the normal anatomy but because understanding it is essential to surgical management. Special radiographs of temporal bones, with areas of interest emphasised by radio-opaque materials have been employed to help clarify the normal radiographic appearances.

Finally, there is no substitute for regular dissection of the temporal bone as a way to full understanding of the subject.

Orientation of pictures

In order to make orientation clearer,'compass bearings' have been placed on several illustrations:

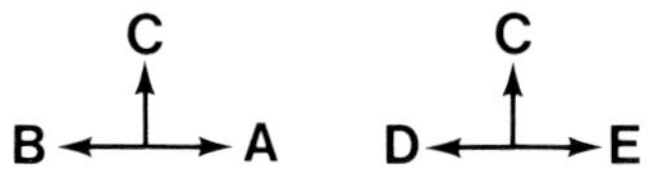

A = Anterior
B = Posterior
C = Superior
D = Medial
E = Lateral

Radiographs

An attempt has been made to clarify the radiographs of the dried temporal bones by adding radio-opaque material to the internal auditory meatus and canal, and to the tympanic annulus.

1

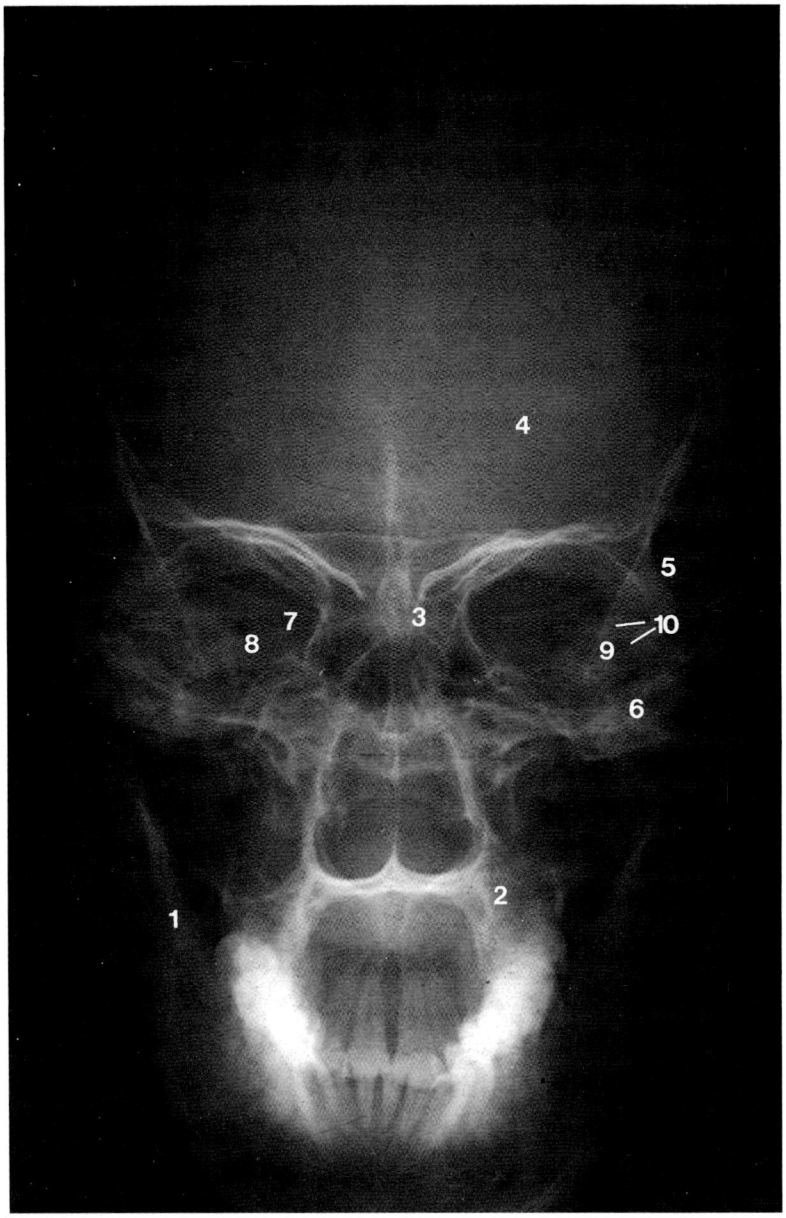

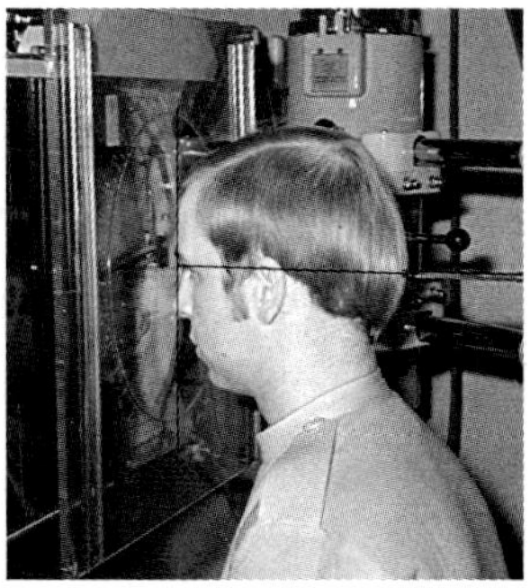

Postero-anterior radiographic position

1 Postero-anterior radiograph of the skull
2 Anterior view of the skull

1 Mandible	7 Internal auditory canal
2 Maxilla	8 Cochlea
3 Nasal bones	9 Vestibule
4 Frontal bone	10 Superior and lateral semi-circular canals
5 Temporal bone	11 Sphenoid bone (greater wing)
6 Zygomatic bone	12 Superior orbital fissure

2

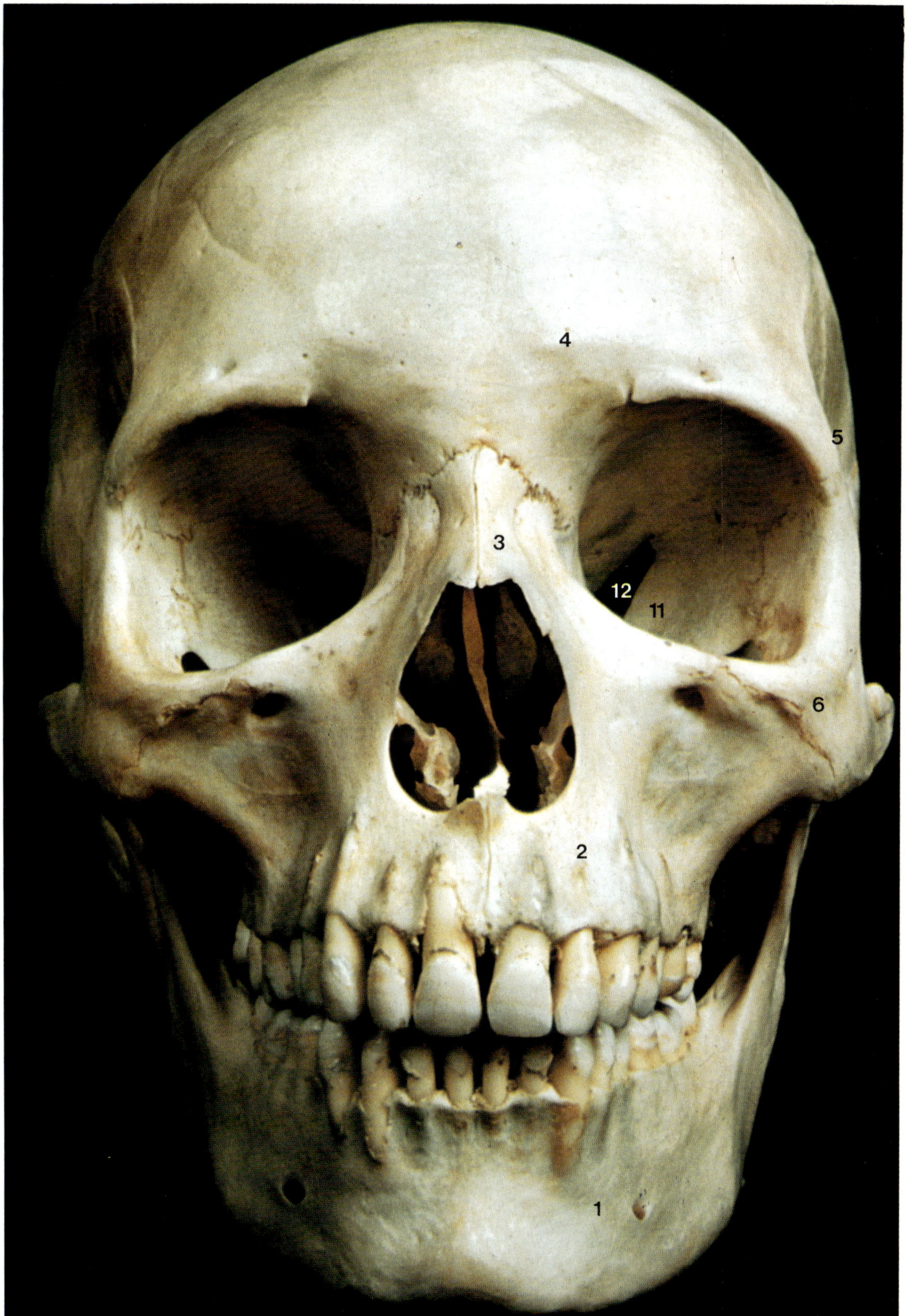

3

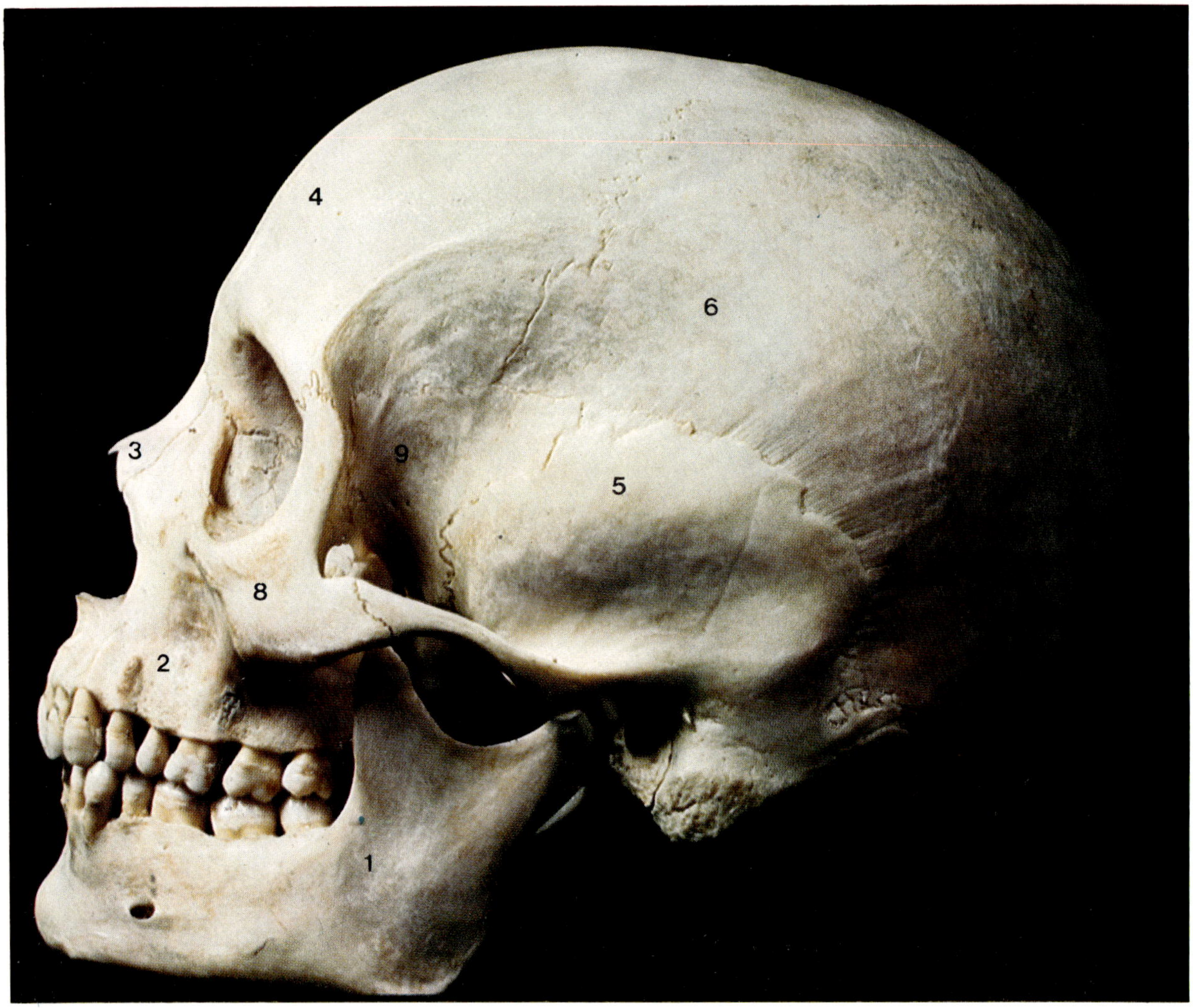

3 Lateral view of skull

1 Mandible
2 Maxilla
3 Nasal bones
4 Frontal bone
5 Temporal bone
6 Parietal bone
7 Occipital bone
8 Zygomatic bone
9 Sphenoid bone

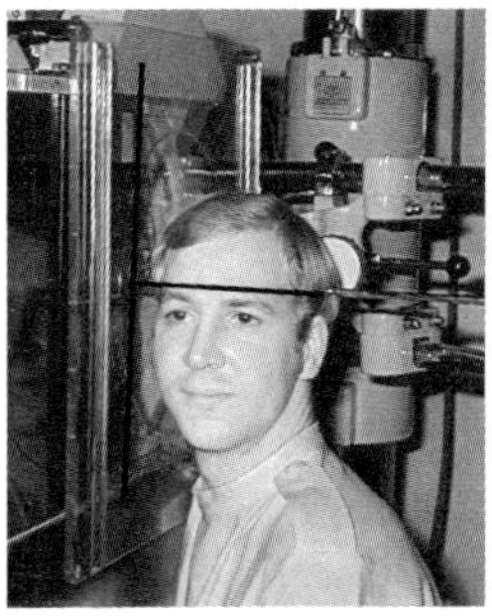

Lateral radiographic position

4

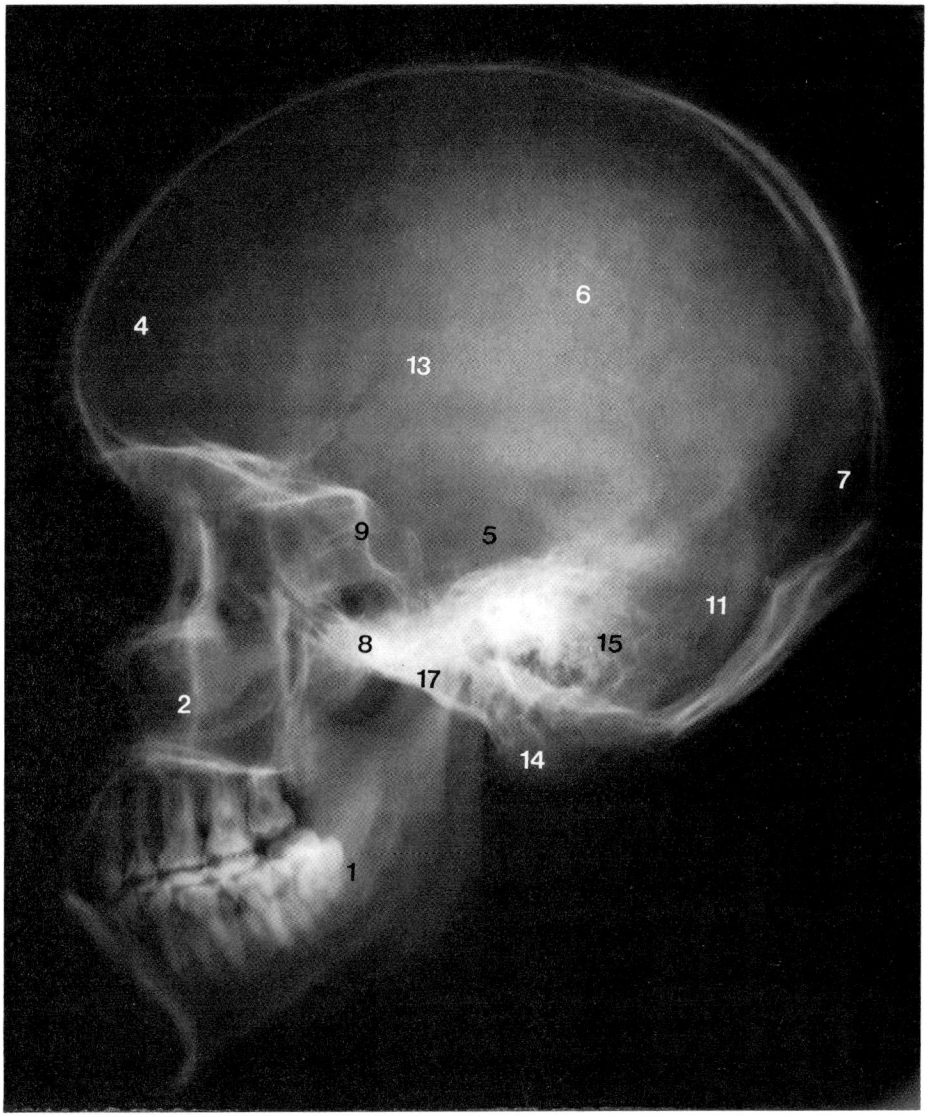

4 Lateral radiograph

10 Tympomastoid suture
11 Parietomastoid suture
12 Sphenosquamosal suture
13 Squamous suture
14 Mastoid process
15 Mastoid air cells
16 External auditory meatus
17 Condylar process of the mandible

5

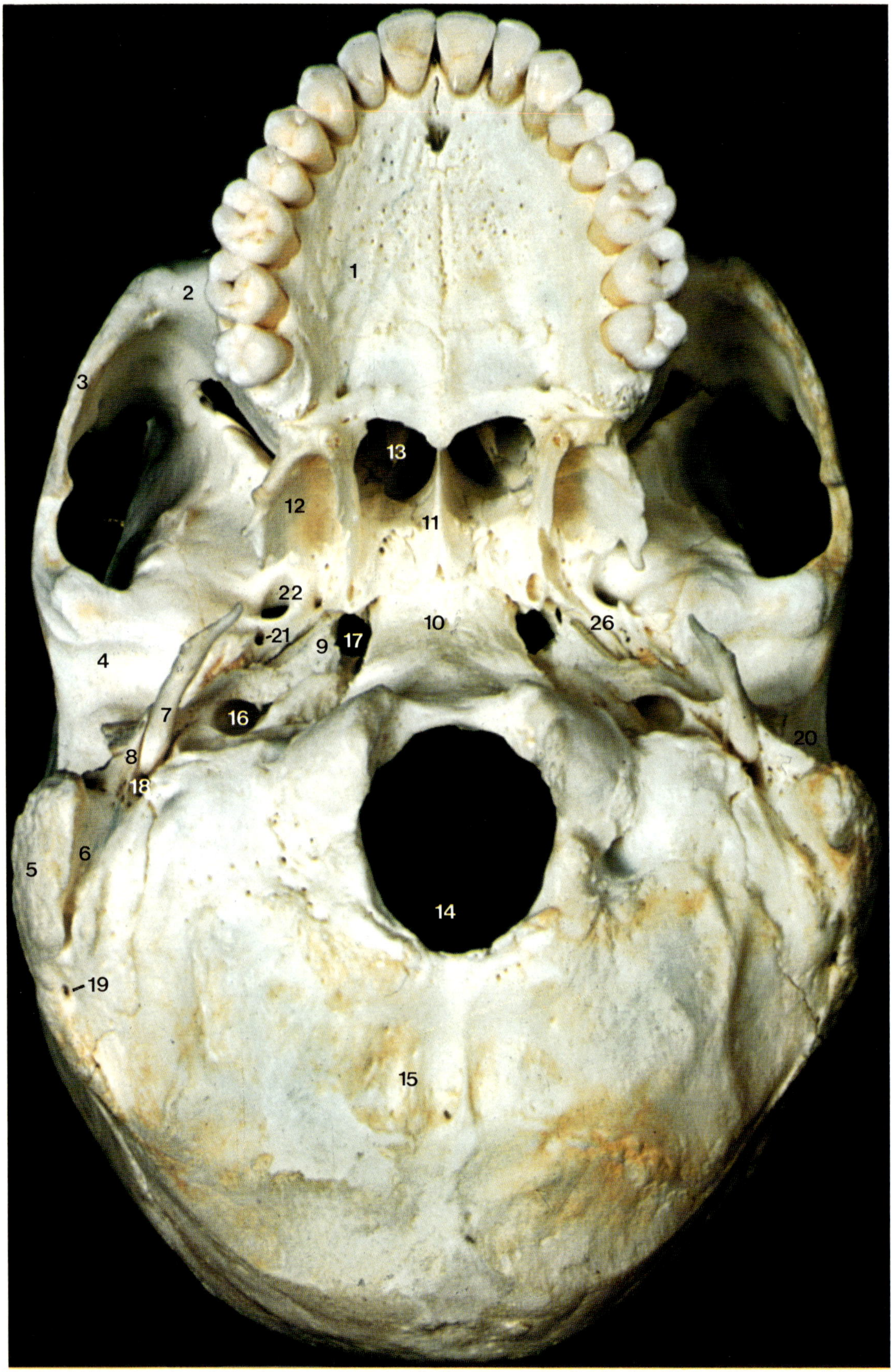

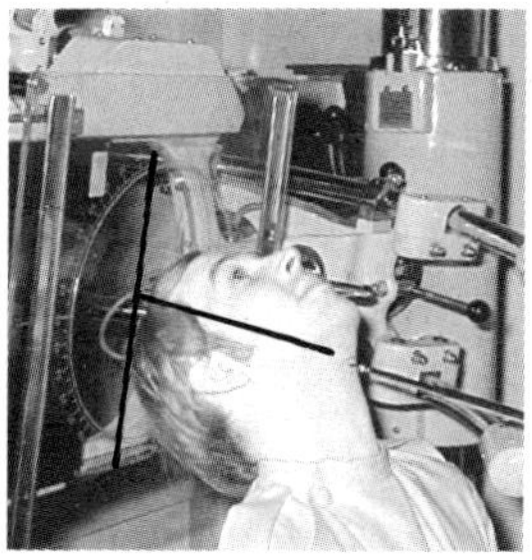

Submento-vertical radiographic position

5 Base of skull (mandible removed)
6 Submento-vertical radiograph

6

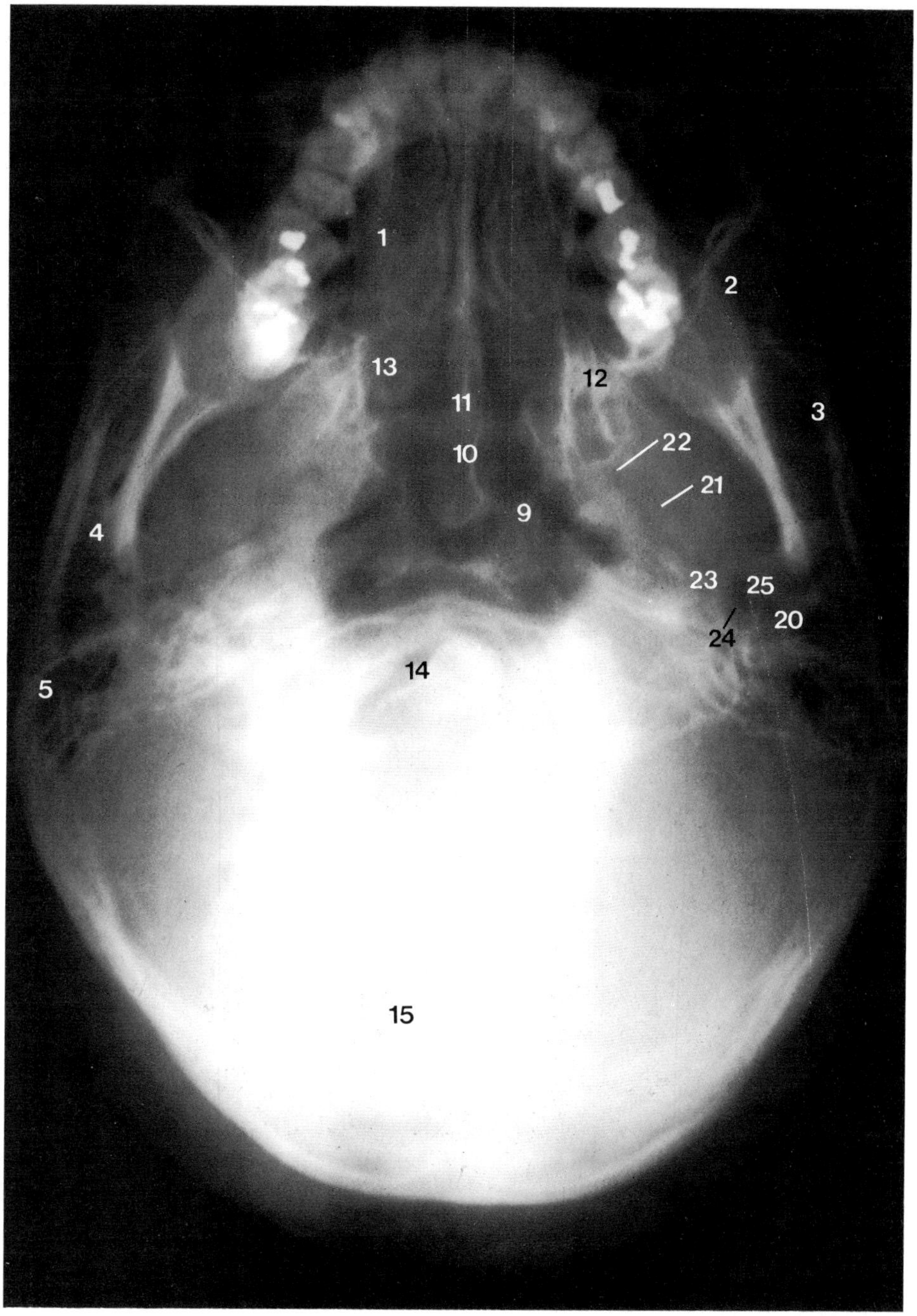

1 Palatine process of the maxilla
2 Lateral wall of the maxilla
3 Zygomatic arch
4 Mandibular fossa
5 Mastoid process
6 Digastric groove
7 Styloid process
8 Styloid process sheath
9 Petrous temporal apex
10 Sphenoid body
11 Vomer
12 Lateral pterygoid plate
13 Posterior nares
14 Foramen magnum
15 Occipital bone
16 Carotid canal
17 Foramen lacerum
18 Stylomastoid foramen
19 Mastoid emissary vein foramen
20 External auditory meatus
21 Foramen spinosum
22 Foramen ovale
23 Bony eustachian tube
24 Middle ear cavity
25 Ossicles (malleus and incus superimposed)
26 Edge of tegmen tympani separating the petrotympanic and petro-squamous sutures

7

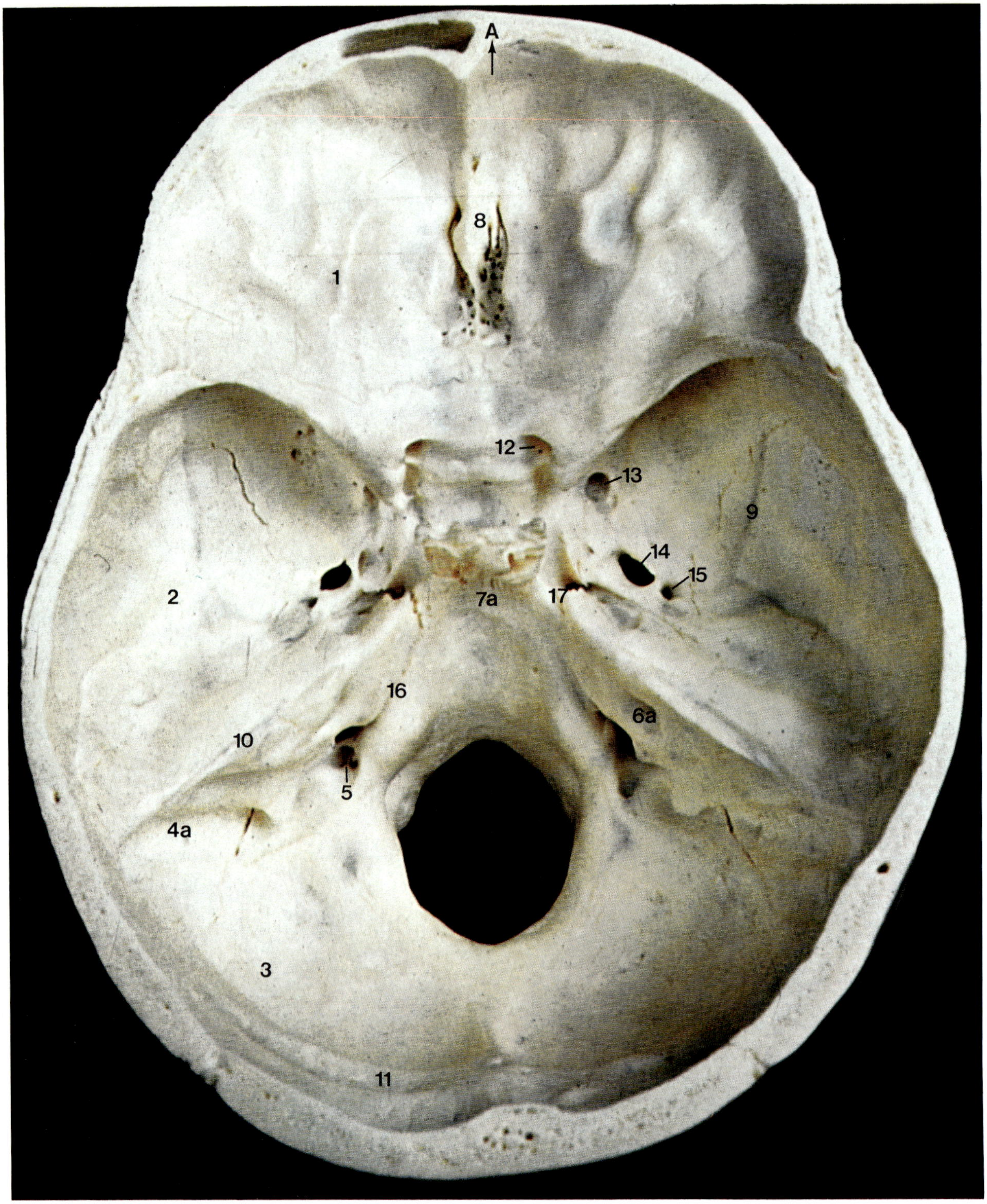

7 Base of dried skull from above

8

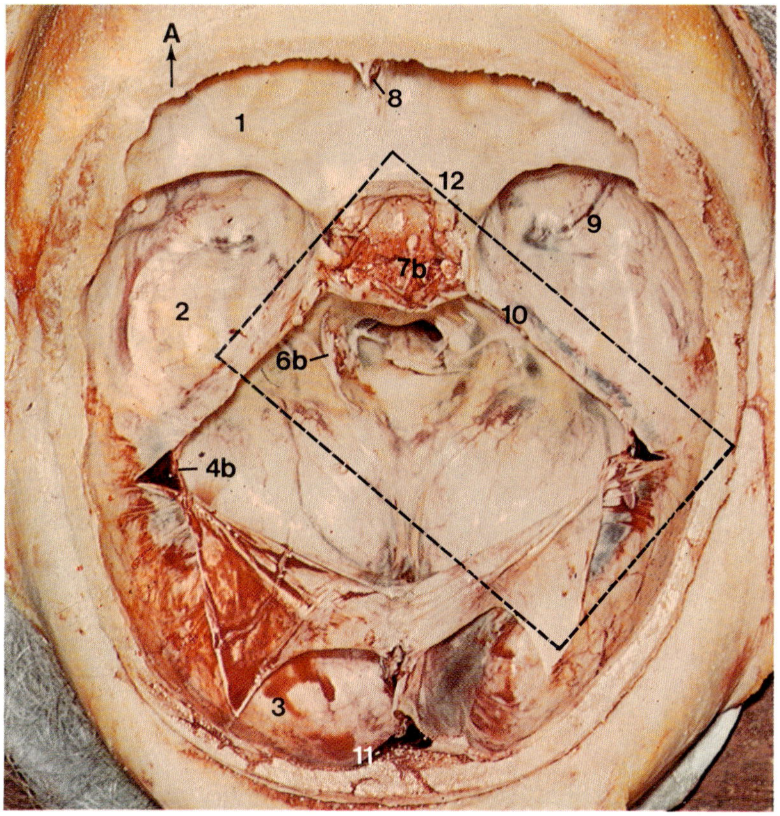

8 Base of skull from above after removal of the brain

1 Anterior cranial fossa
2 Middle cranial fossa
3 Posterior cranial fossa
4 a) Sigmoid sulcus
b) Sigmoid sinus
5 Jugular foramen
6 a) Internal auditory meatus
b) Vestibulocochlear and facial nerves at the meatus
7 a) Dorsum sellae
b) Pituitary fossa
8 Crista galli
9 Middle meningeal vessels and groove
10 Superior petrosal sinus and groove
11 Transverse sinus and groove
12 Optic nerve and optic foramen
13 Foramen rotundum
14 Foramen ovale
15 Foramen spinosum
16 Inferior petrosal sinus
17 Petrous tip

Note: The area within the rectangle is shown in greater detail on page 30.

9

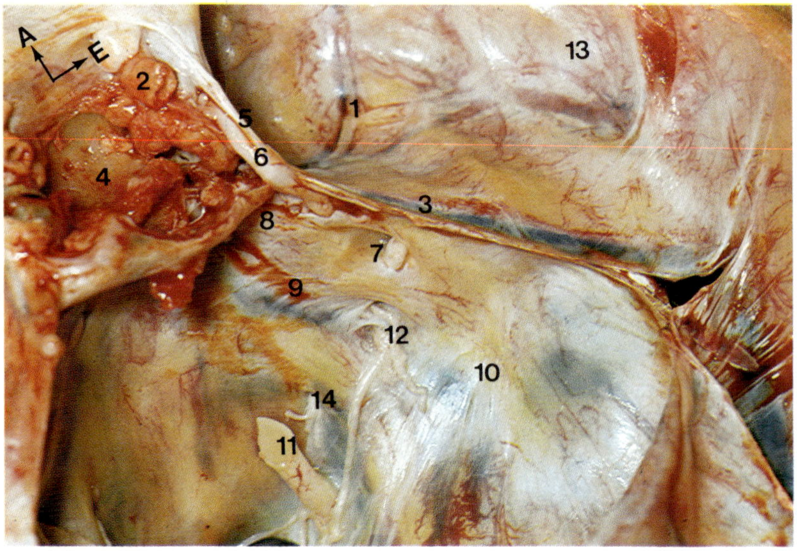

9 Superior surface of right temporal bone in a skull base with dura attached

10

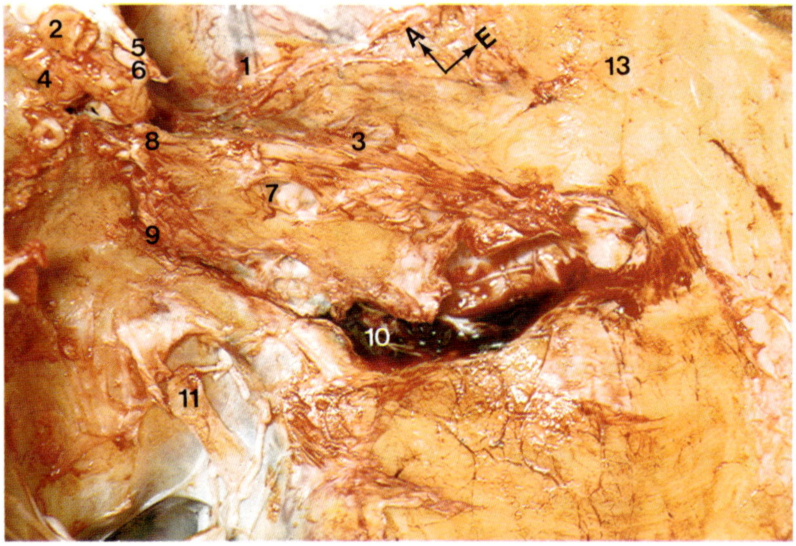

10 As above but with the dura stripped

1 Middle meningeal artery
2 Internal carotid artery
3 Superior petrosal sinus
4 Pituitary fossa
5 Petro-clinoid ligament
6 Oculomotor (III) cranial nerve
7 Internal auditory meatus with VII and VIII cranial nerves
8 Petrous bone apex
9 Inferior petrosal sinus
10 Superior bulb of the internal jugular vein
11 Vertebral artery
12 Cranial nerves IX, X, XI
13 Middle cranial fossa
14 Hypoglossal nerve (XII)

11 Superior view of right temporal bone

11

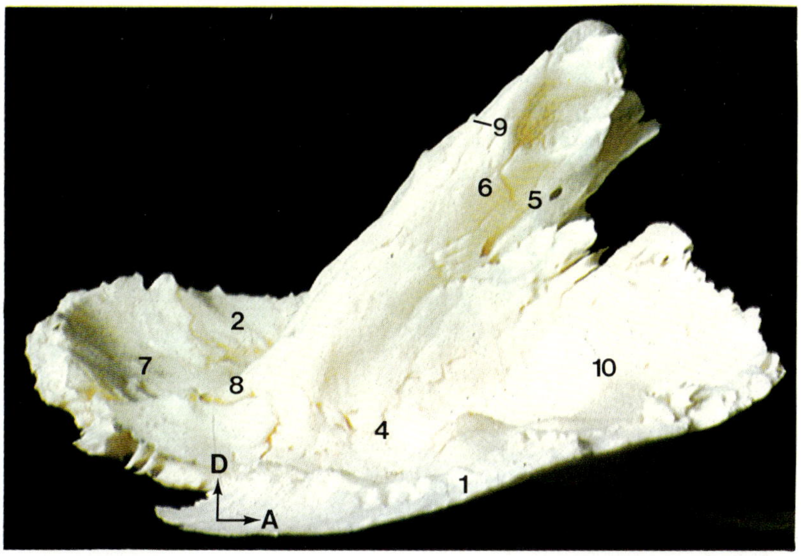

12 Occipito-mental radiograph of dry temporal bone

12

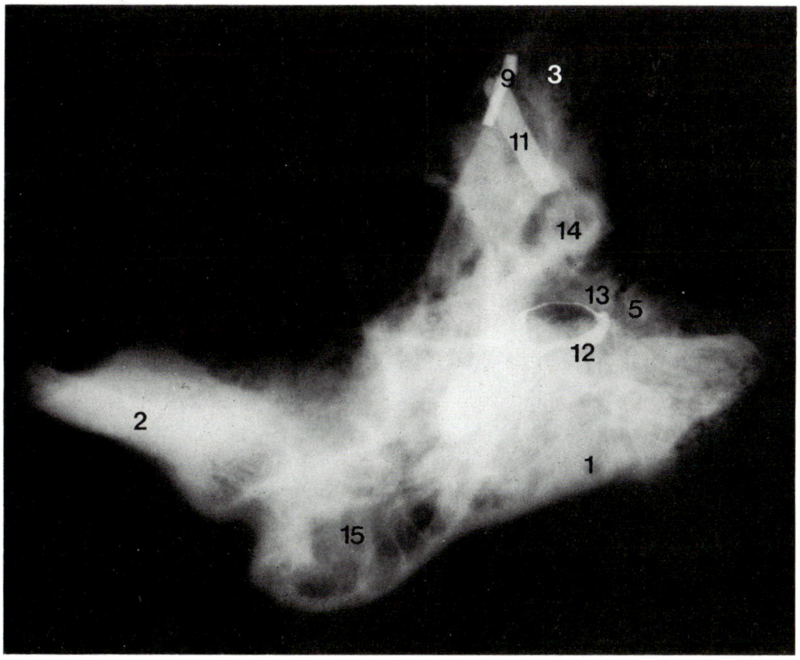

1 Squamous part
2 Mastoid part
3 Petrous tip
4 Petro-squamous fissure
5 Tegmen tympani (removed on radiography)
6 Arcuate eminence
7 Sigmoid sulcus
8 Superior petrosal sulcus
9 Internal auditory meatus
10 Cerebral impressions
11 Internal auditory canal
12 Tympanic annulus
13 Incudo-malleus complex
14 Cochlear turns
15 Mastoid air cells

13

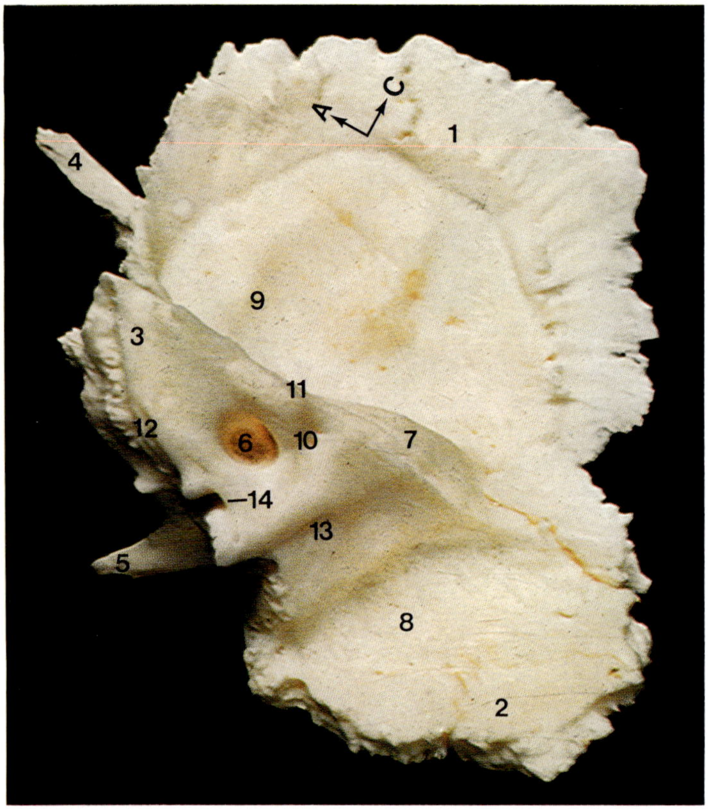

13 Medial view of right temporal bone

1 Squamous temporal part
2 Mastoid part
3 Petrous part
4 Zygomatic process
5 Styloid process
6 Internal auditory canal
7 Arcuate eminence (mainly superior semicircular canal)
8 Sigmoid sulcus
9 Cerebral convolution impressions
10 Subarcuate fossa (small veins)
11 Superior petrosal sulcus
12 Inferior petrosal sulcus
13 Vestibular aqueduct (external opening for the endolymphatic sac and duct)
14 Cochlear canaliculus (external opening for the perilymphatic 'duct')

14

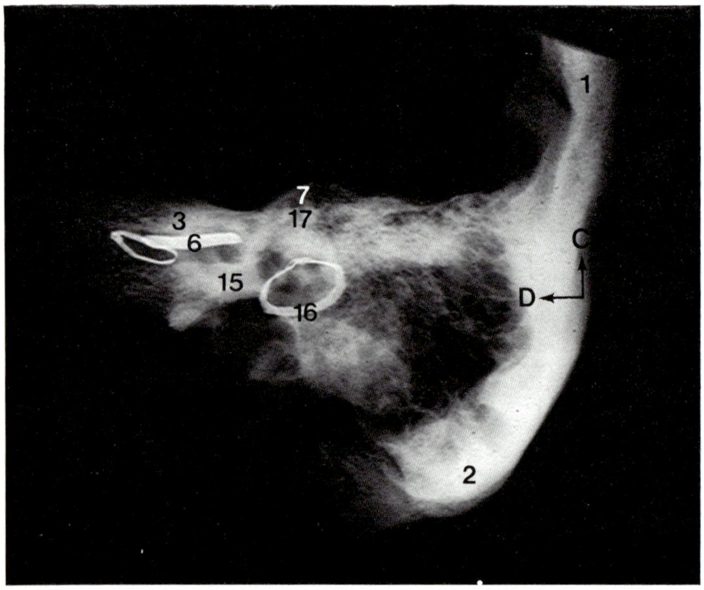

14 Stenver's view of a dry temporal bone

15 Cochlea
16 Tympanic ring
17 Superior semicircular canal

15

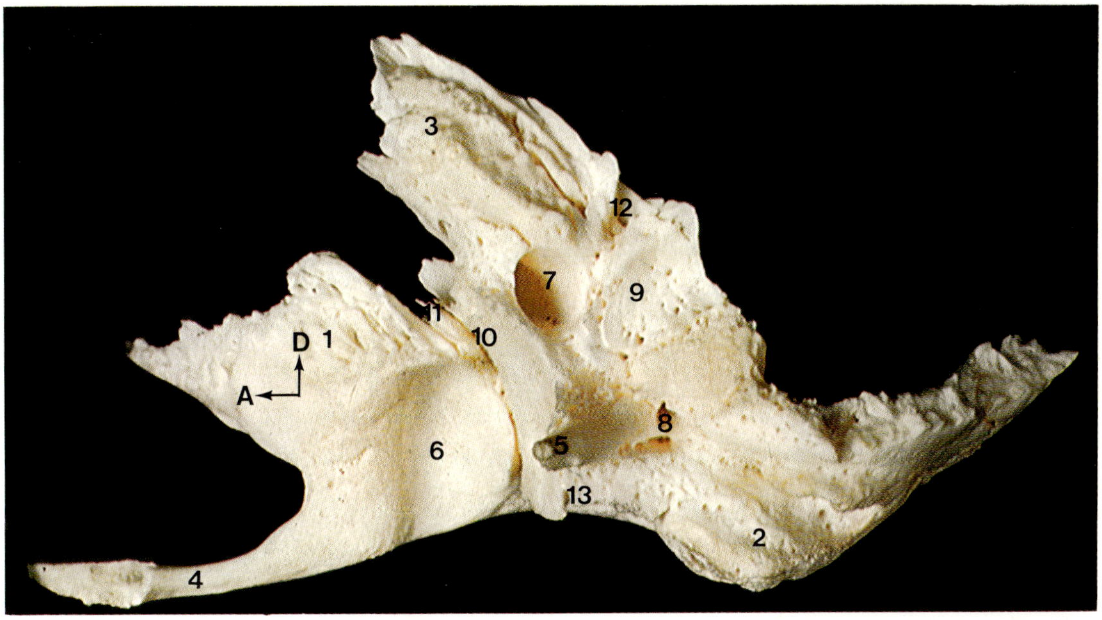

15 Inferior view of right temporal bone

16

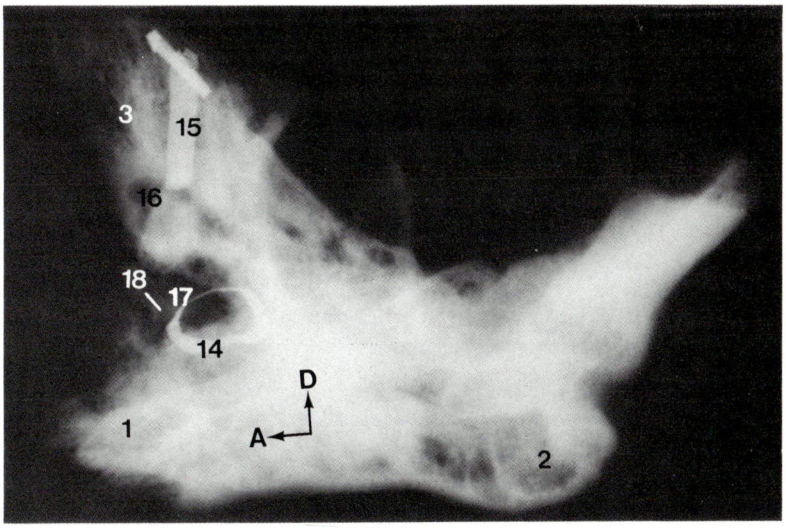

16 Submento-vertical radiograph of a dry temporal bone

1 Squamous part
2 Mastoid part
3 Petrous part
4 Zygomatic process
5 Styloid process
6 Mandibular fossa
7 Carotid canal
8 Stylomastoid foramen
9 Jugular fossa
10 Squamotympanic fissure
11 Downturned edge of tegmen tympani
12 Cochlear canaliculus
13 External auditory meatus
14 Tympanic annulus
15 Internal auditory canal and meatus
16 Cochlea
17 Middle ear (without tegmen)
18 Head of malleus

17

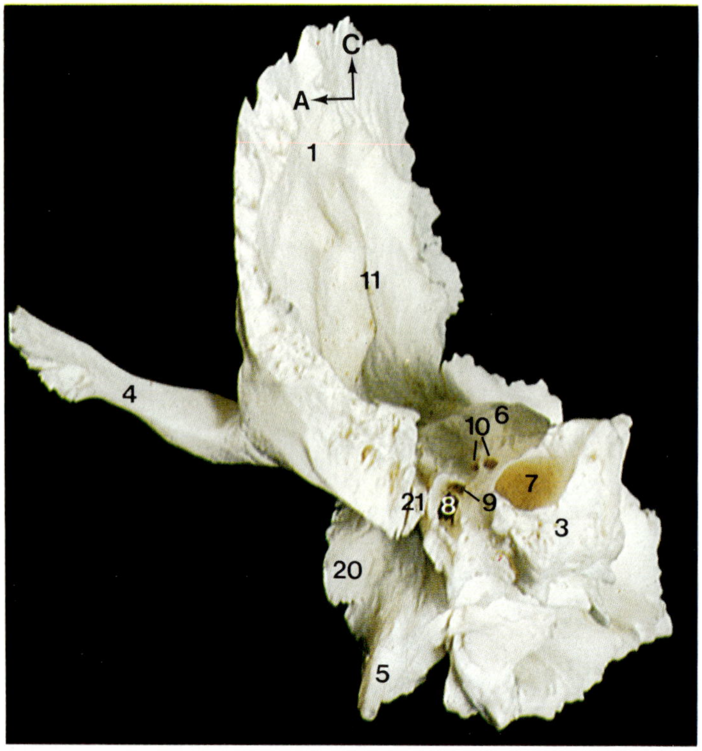

17 Anterior view of right temporal bone

18

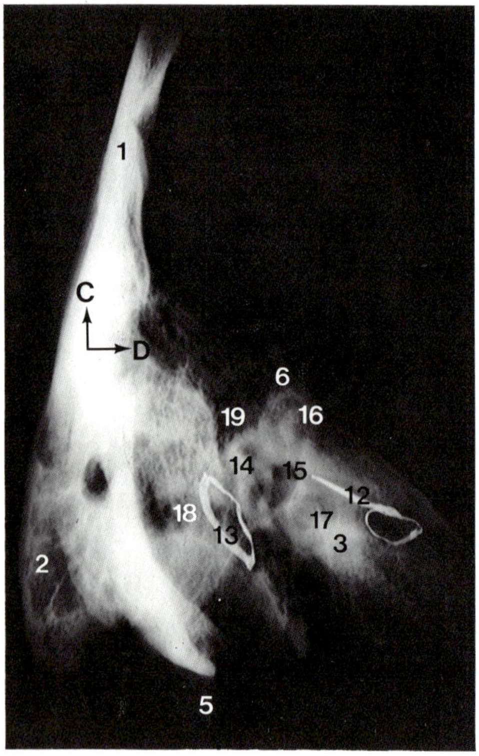

18 Townes radiograph of dry temporal bone

1 Squamous part
2 Mastoid part
3 Petrous part
4 Zygomatic process
5 Styloid process and sheath
6 Arcuate eminence
7 Carotid canal
8 Eustachian tube semicanal
9 Tensor tympani muscle semicanal
10 Greater and lesser petrosal grooves
11 Vascular sulci

19

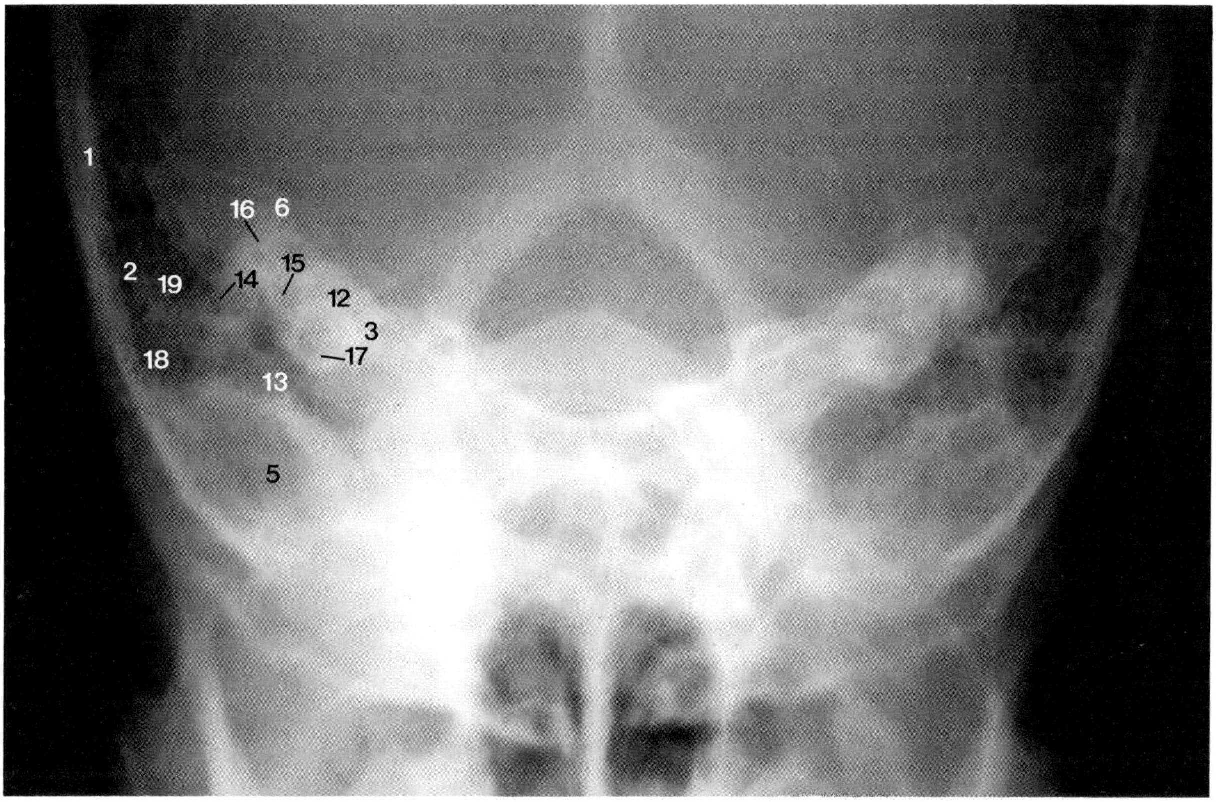

19 Townes (30° fronto-occipital) radiograph

12 Internal auditory canal and meatus
13 Tympanic annulus
14 Heads of incus and malleus
15 Vestibule
16 Superior semicircular canal
17 First turn of the cochlea
18 External auditory canal
19 Mastoid antrum
20 Tympanic part of temporal bone
21 Downturned part of tegmen tympani between the petrous and squamous parts of the temporal bone

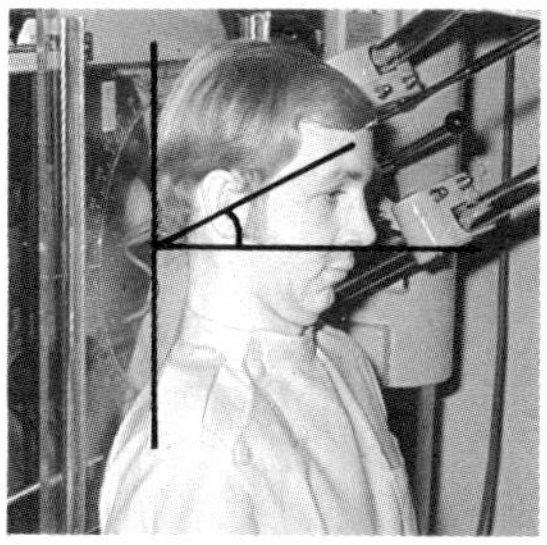

Townes (30° fronto-occipital) radiographic position

20

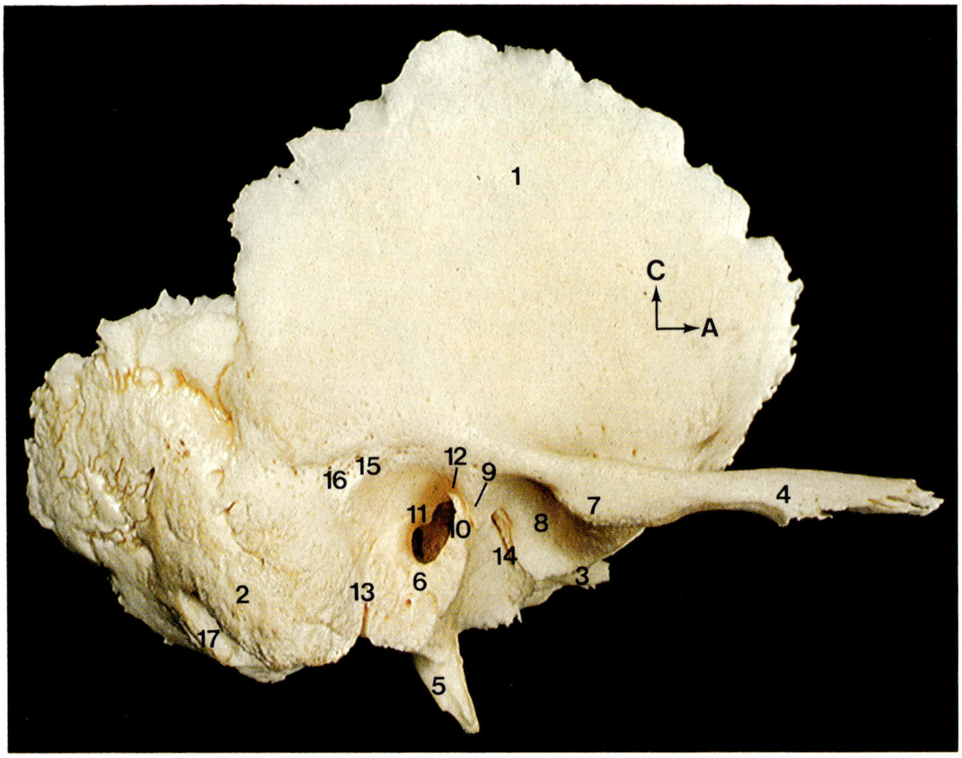

20 Lateral view of right temporal bone

21

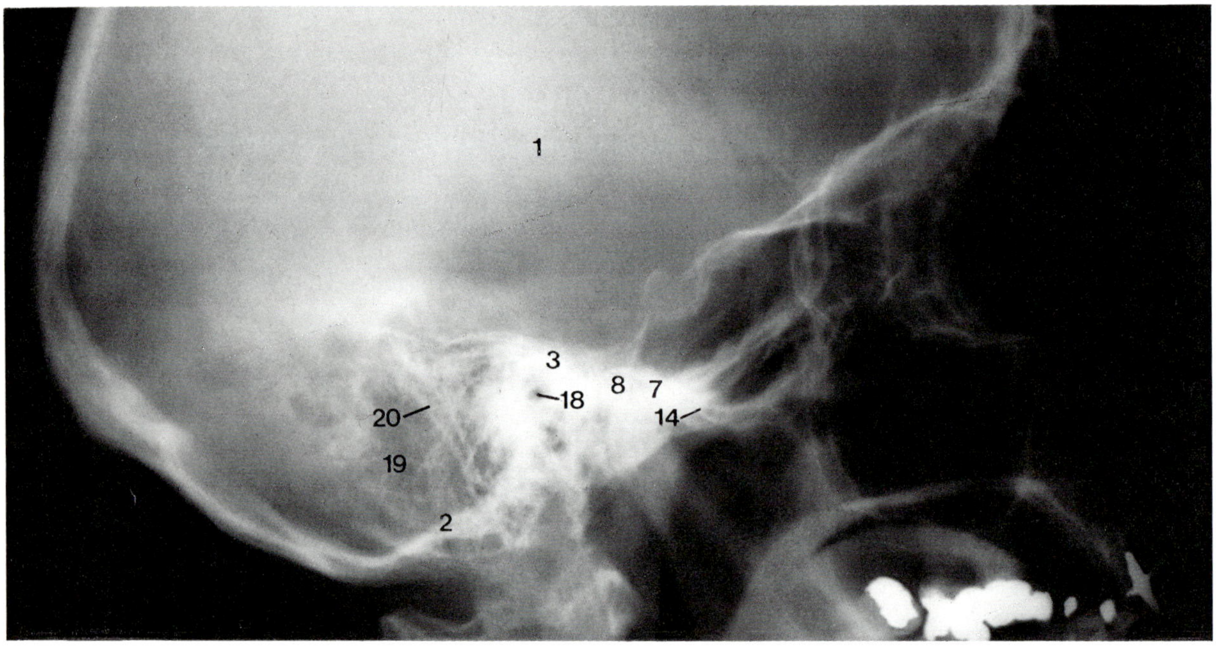

21 Lateral radiograph

22

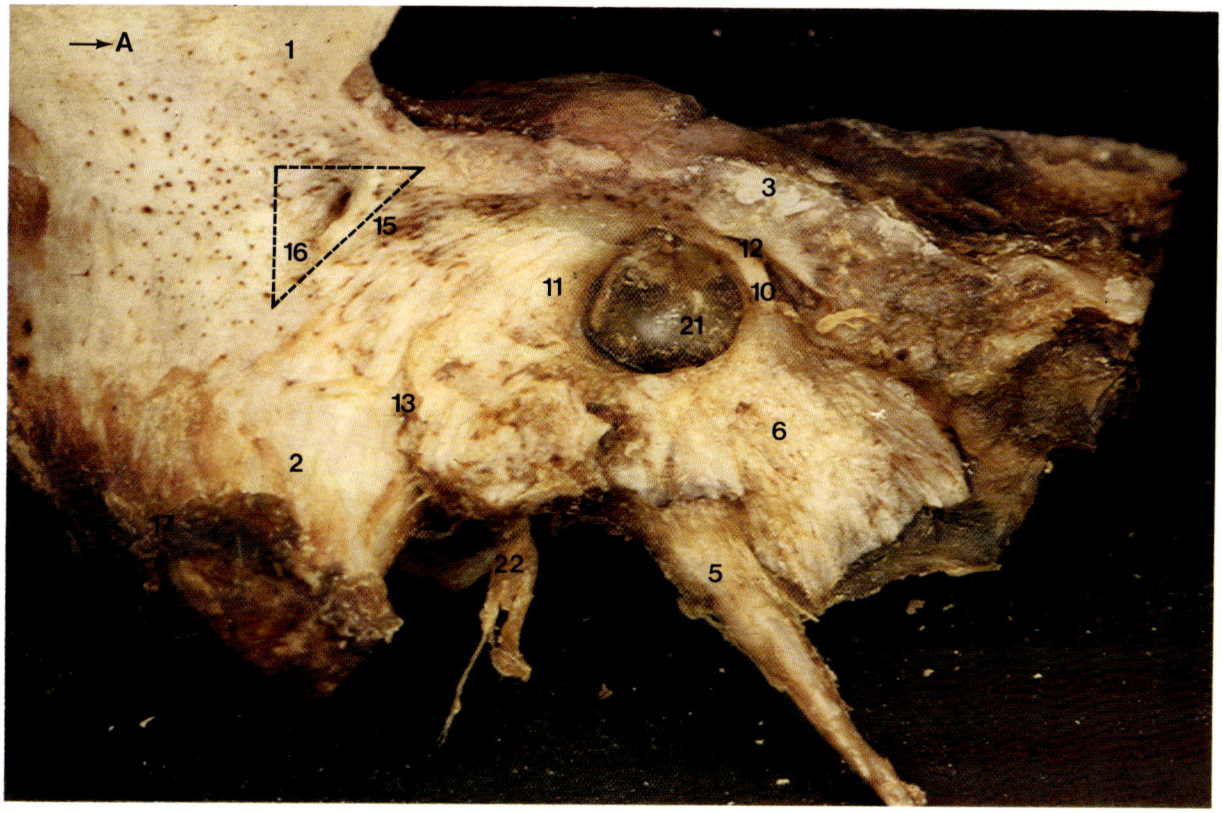

22 Lateral view of right temporal bone with the anterior wall of the external auditory canal removed with the zygomatic process

1 Squamous part
2 Mastoid part
3 Petrous part
4 Zygomatic process
5 Styloid process and sheath
6 Tympanic part
7 Articular tubercle
8 Mandibular fossa
9 Postglenoid tubercle
10 Anterior border of external auditory canal
11 External auditory canal
12 Squamotympanic fissure
13 Tympanomastoid suture
14 Petrotympanic fissure
15 Suprameatal spine
16 Suprameatal triangle
17 Digastric groove
18 Superimposed internal and external auditory canals
19 Mastoid air cells
20 Lateral sinus plate
21 Tympanic membrane
22 Facial nerve

23

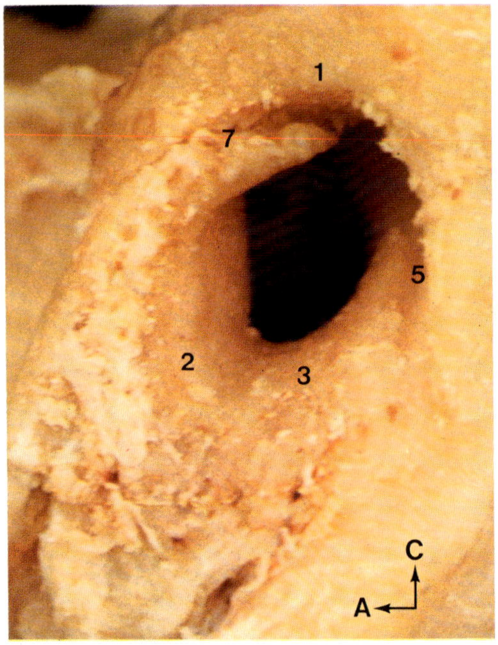

23 **Bony external auditory meatus**

24

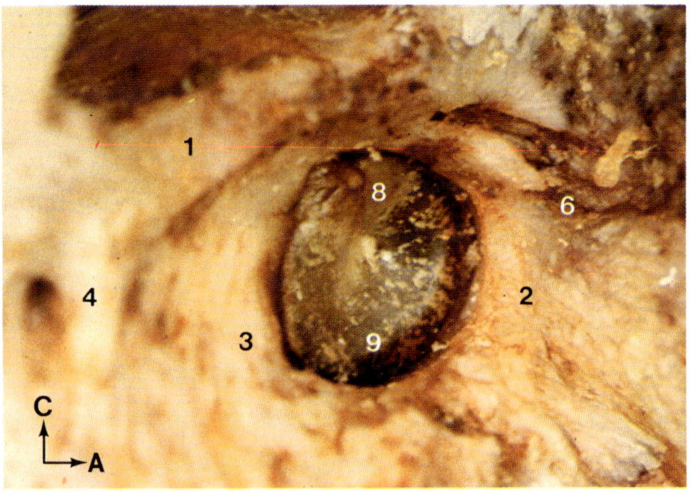

24 External auditory canal with the anterior wall removed

1 Squamous part
2 Tympanic part
3 External auditory canal
4 Suprameatal spine
5 Tympanomastoid suture
6 Petrotympanic fissure
7 Tympanosquamous suture
8 Lateral process of malleus
9 Tympanic membrane

25

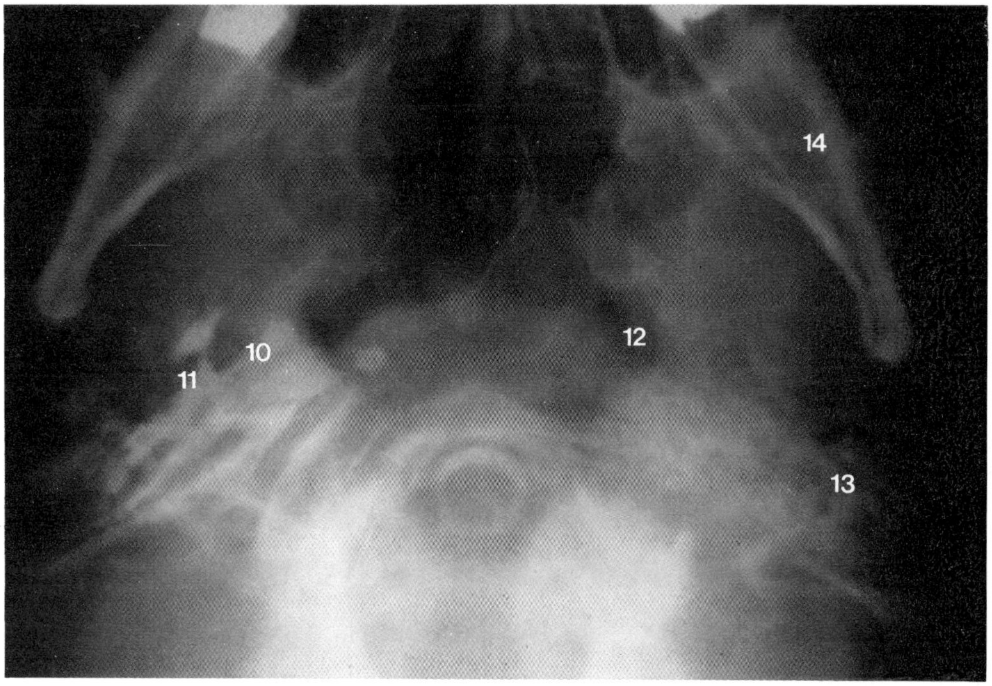

25 Submento-vertical radiograph

26

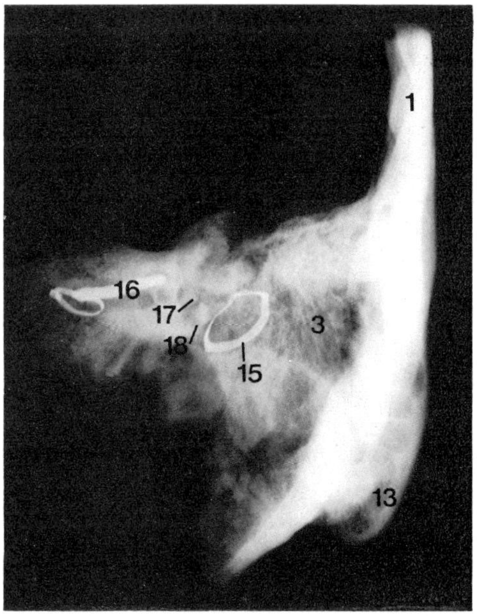

26 Postero-anterior view of a dry temporal bone (tegmen removed)

10 Eustachian tube
11 Middle ear
12 Lateral recess of nasopharynx
13 Mastoid air cells
14 Mandible
15 Tympanic annulus
16 Internal auditory canal and meatus
17 Vestibule
18 Posterior semicircular canal

27

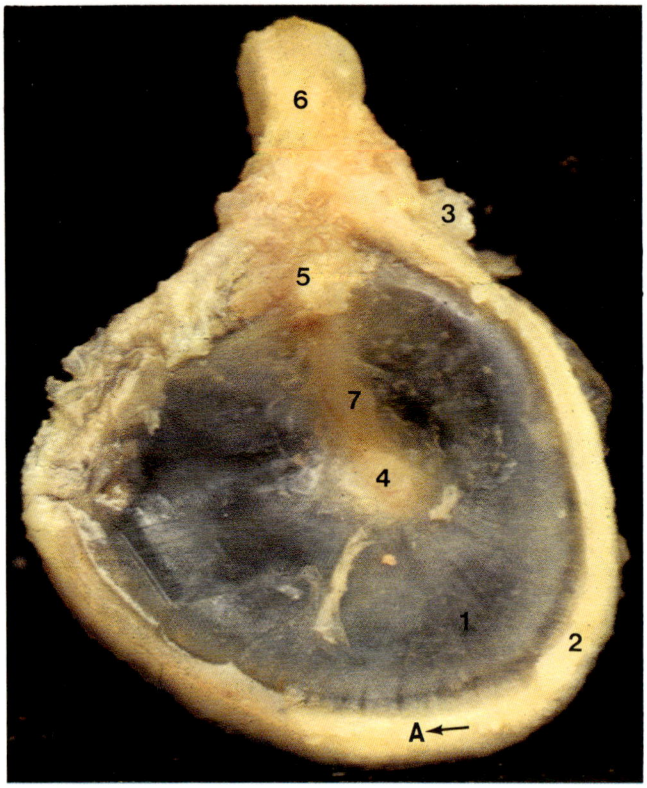

27 Lateral surface of tympanic membrane

28

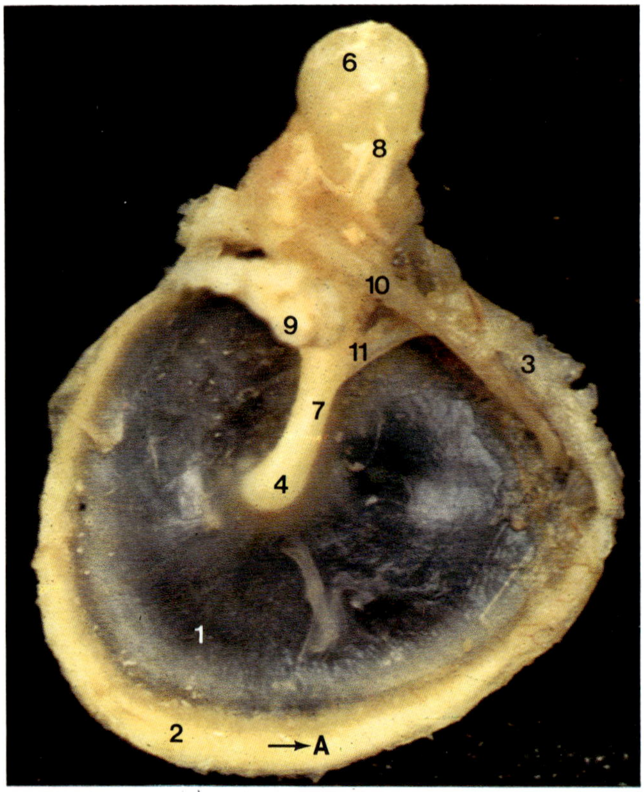

28 Medial surface of tympanic membrane

29

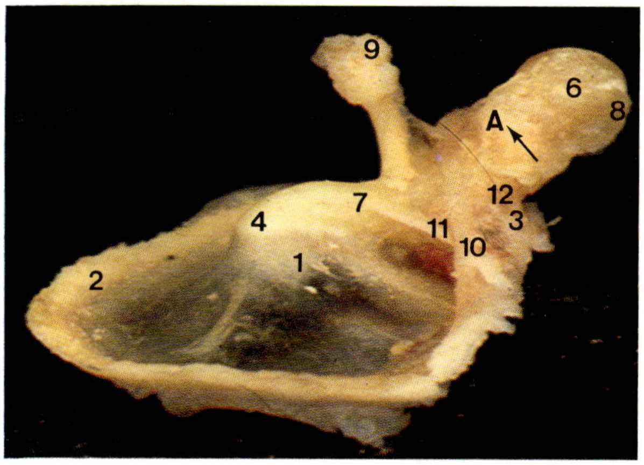

29 Side view of tympanic membrane

30

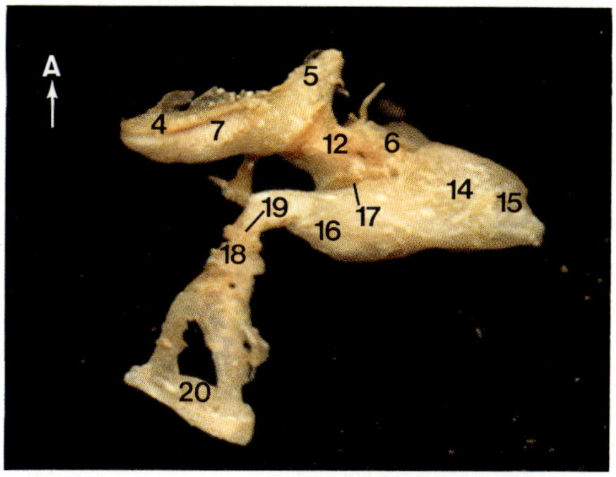

30 Postero-inferior view of ossicular chain

31

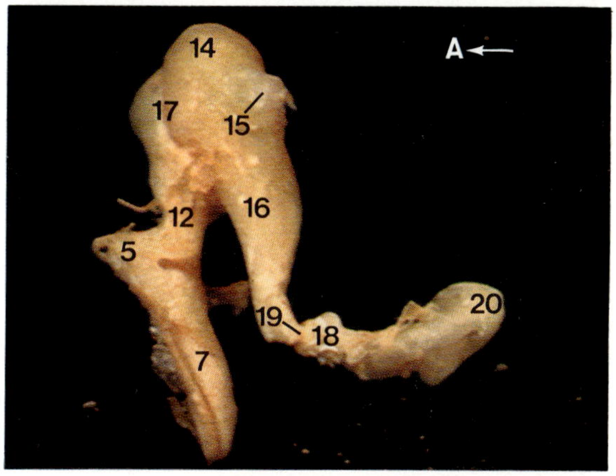

31 Posterior view of ossicular chain

32

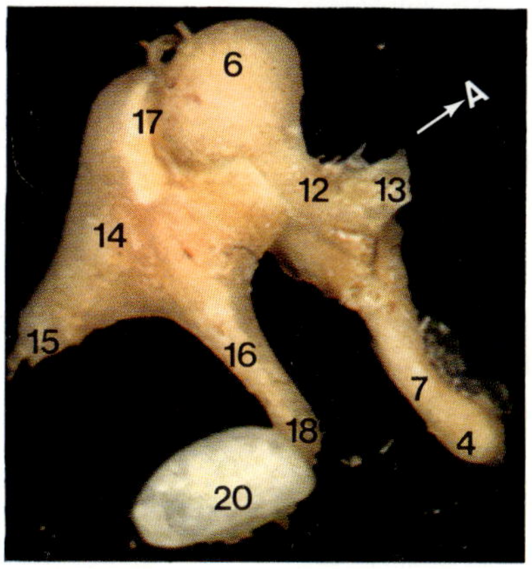

32 Medial view of ossicular chain

1 Tympanic membrane
2 Tympanic ring (annulus fibrosus)
3 Remnant of external auditory canal lining
4 Umbo
5 Lateral process of malleus
6 Head of malleus
7 Handle of malleus
8 Articular surface of malleus with incus
9 Tensor tympani tendon
10 Chorda tympani
11 Stria membrana tympani anticus
12 Neck of malleus
13 Anterior process of malleus
14 Body of incus
15 Short process of incus
16 Long process of incus
17 Incudo-malleolar joint
18 Incudo-stapedial joint
19 Lentiform process
20 Stapes

33

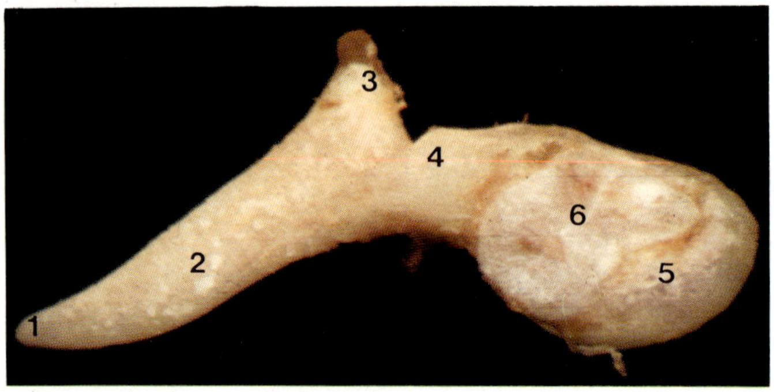

33 Left malleus—posterior view

34

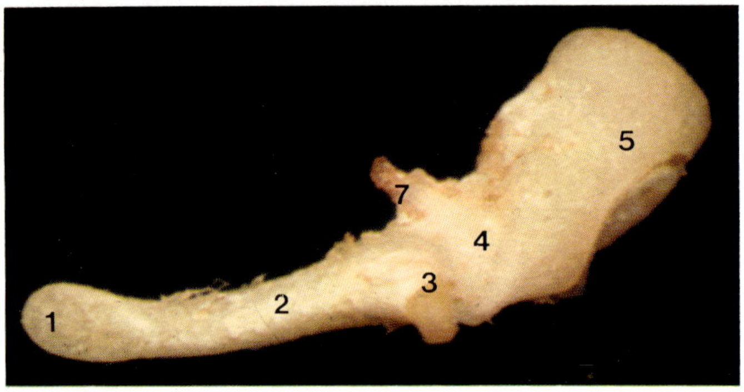

34 Left malleus—lateral view

35

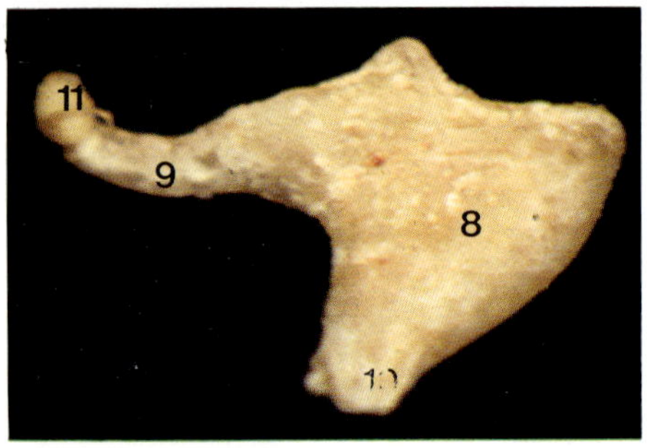

35 Right incus—medial view

36

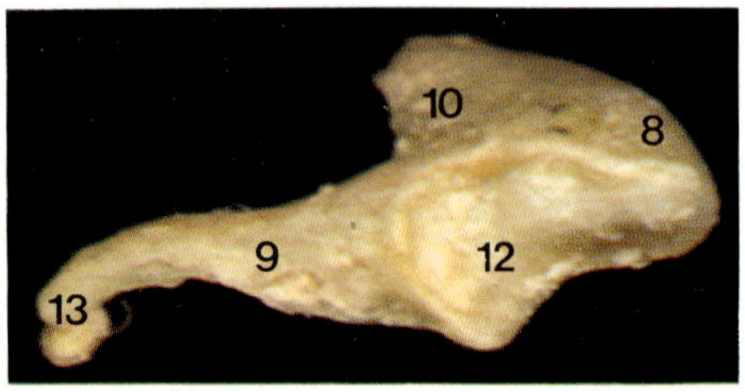

36 Right incus—anterior view

37

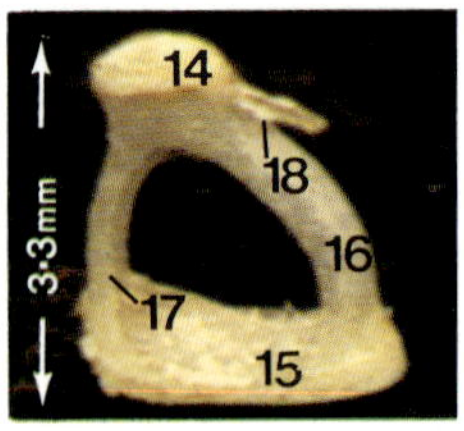

38

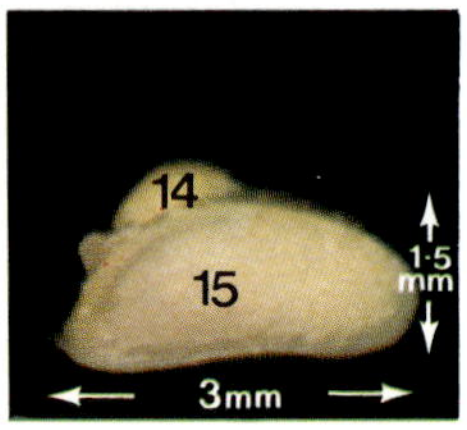

37 Right stapes—superior view
38 Left stapes footplate—medial view

1 Umbo (with flat surface for attachment of the tympanic membrane)
2 Handle of malleus
3 Lateral process of malleus
4 Neck of malleus
5 Head of malleus
6 Articular surface with incus
7 Anterior process of malleus with anterior malleolar ligament
8 Body of incus
9 Long process of incus
10 Short process of incus
11 Articular surface of the lentiform process of incus
12 Articular surface with malleus
13 Lentiform process
14 Head of stapes
15 Footplate of stapes
16 Posterior (curved) crus
17 Anterior (straight) crus
18 Attachment of stapedius tendon to the neck of the stapes

Note: Stapes measurements are average

39

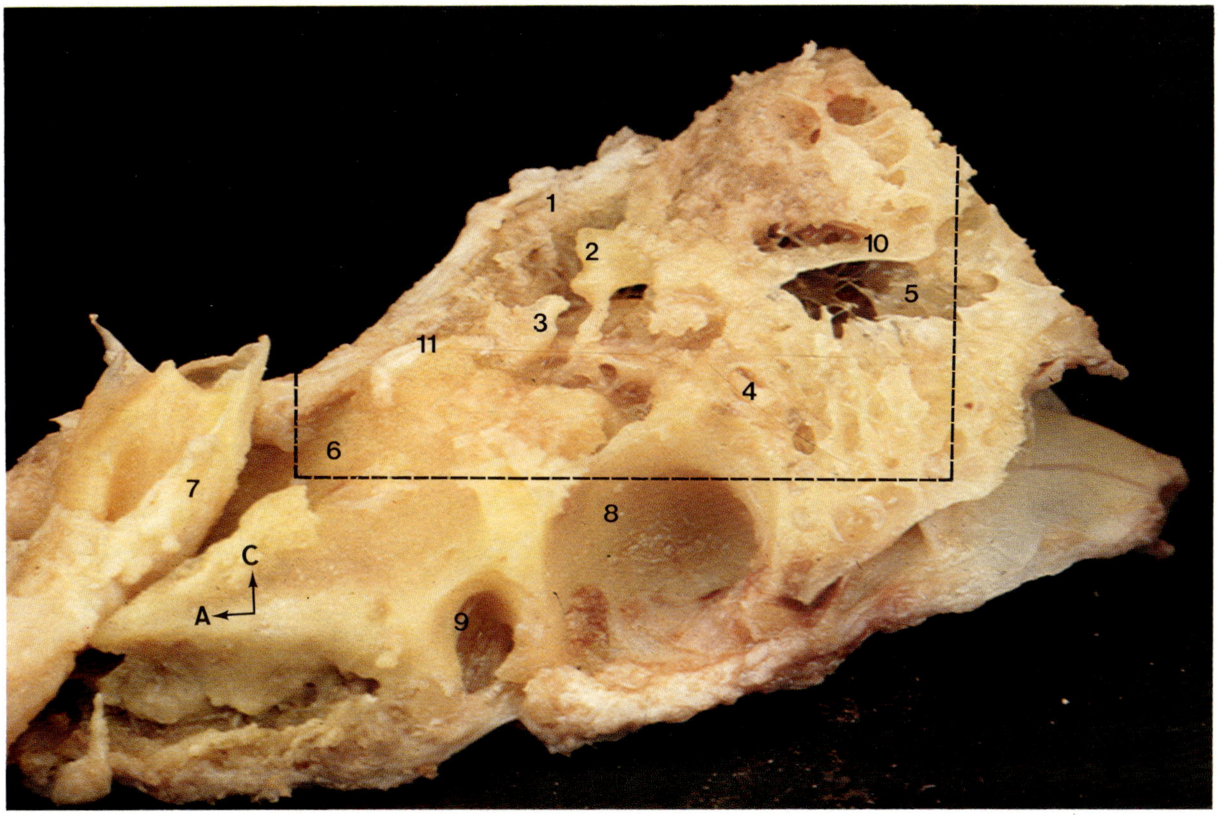

39 Lateral view of the medial wall of the left tympanic cavity

1 Tegmen tympani
2 Body of incus
3 Cochleariform process
4 Facial nerve (vertical protion)
5 Mastoid cavity
6 Eustachian tube (bony portion)
7 Mucosa and cartilage of eustachian tube
8 Jugular fossa
9 Carotid canal
10 Körner's septum
11 Tensor tympani muscle

Note: The area within the rectangle is shown in greater detail on page 30.

40

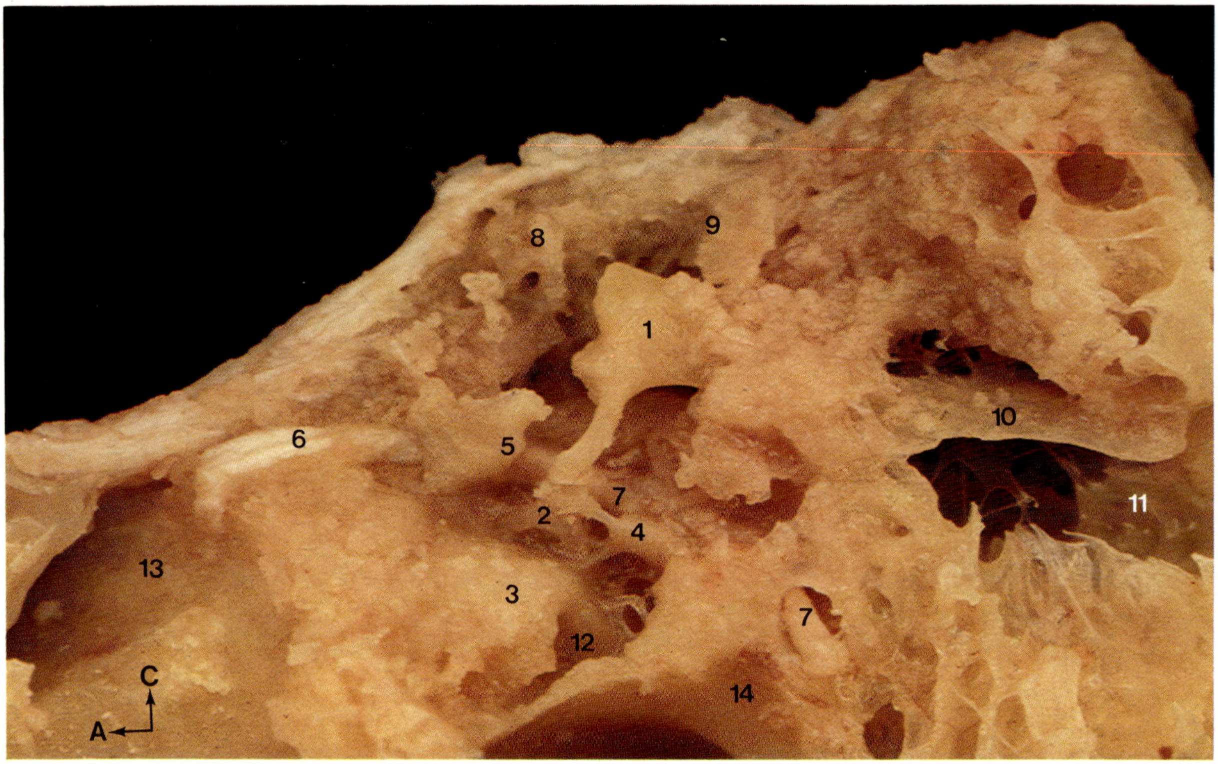

40 Close up of the medial wall of the left tympanic cavity

1 Incus
2 Stapes
3 Promontory
4 Pyramid with stapedius tendon
5 Cochleariform process
6 Tensor tympani muscle
7 Facial nerve
8 Tegmen tympani
9 Aditus
10 Körner's septum
11 Mastoid cavity
12 Round window
13 Bony eustachian tube
14 Jugular fossa

Note: The facial nerve may have no bony covering in its horizontal portion in 20-30 per cent.

41

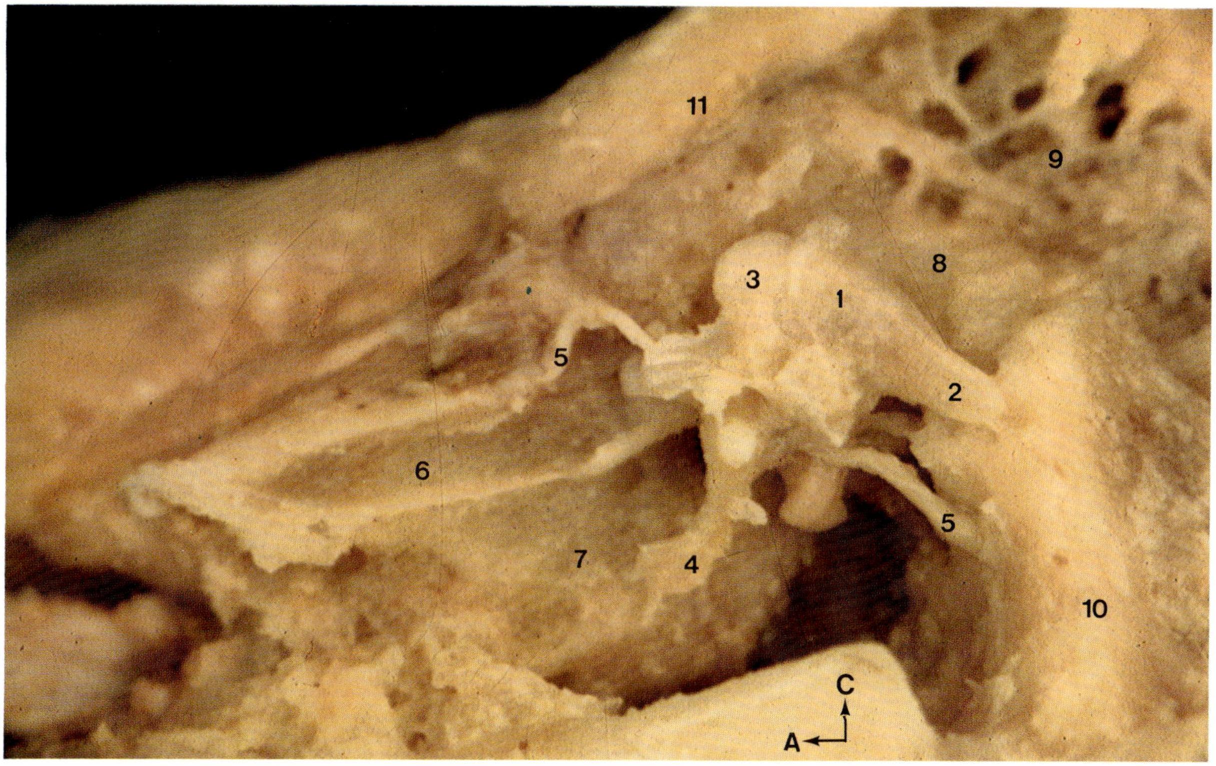

41 Lateral view of medial wall of the left tympanic cavity

1 Body of incus
2 Short process of incus
3 Head of malleus
4 Umbo of malleus (membrane removed)
5 Chorda tympani
6 Semicanal for tensor tympani muscle (muscle removed)
7 Promontory
8 Lateral semicircular canal
9 Antrum of mastoid
10 Posterior canal wall (bridge) removed
11 Tegmen tympani

Note: a) The short process of the incus is vital in assessing the situation of the facial nerve lying medially.
b) The bridge is the area removed in doing any radical form of mastoidectomy

42

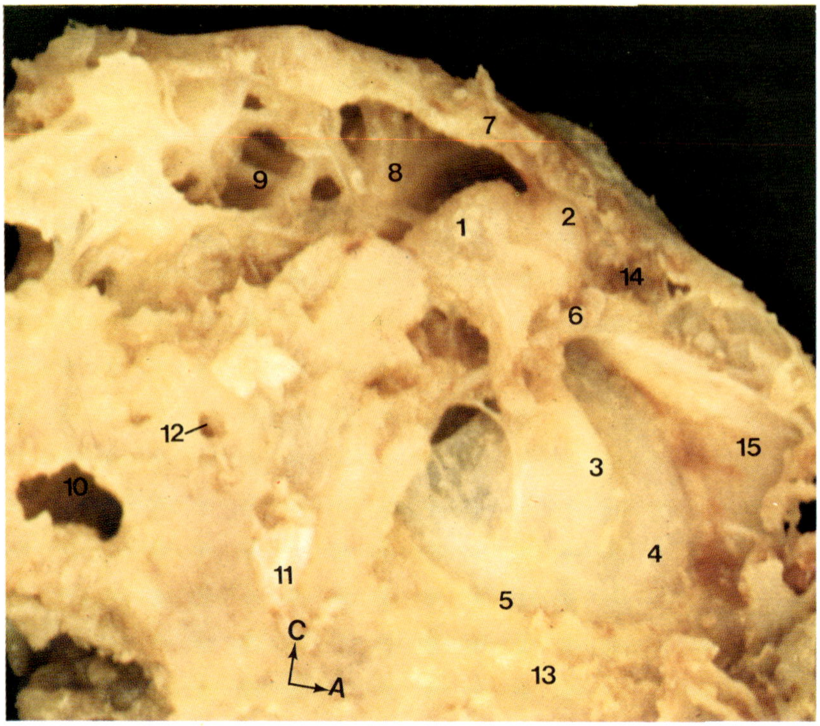

42 Medial view of the lateral wall of the right tympanic cavity

1 Body of incus
2 Head of malleus
3 Umbo of malleus
4 Tympanic membrane (limbus)
5 Tympanic ring (annulus)
6 Chorda tympani entering petro-tympanic fissure
7 Tegmen tympani
8 Aditus
9 Antrum
10 Mastoid cavity
11 Facial nerve (cut)
12 Lateral semicircular canal
13 Hypotympanum
14 Epitympanum
15 Eustachian tube

43

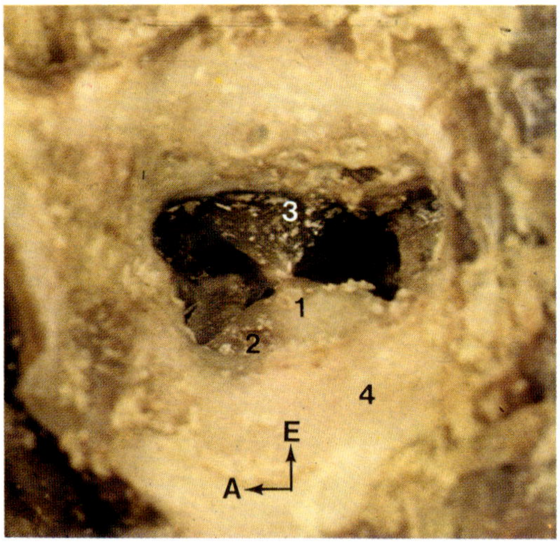

43 Inferior view of tympanic cavity through the jugular fossa

1 Inferior surface of promontory
2 Round window membrane
3 Tympanic membrane (very indrawn)
4 Wall of jugular fossa

44 Superior view of tympanic cavity (tegmen removed)

44

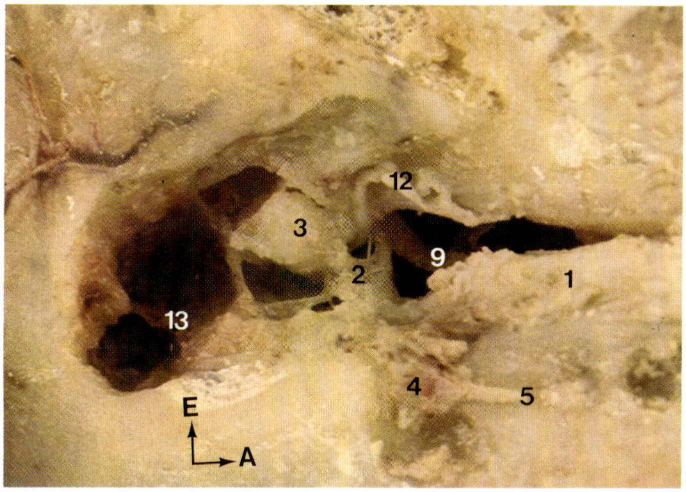

45 Superior view of left tympanic cavity (tegmen removed)

45

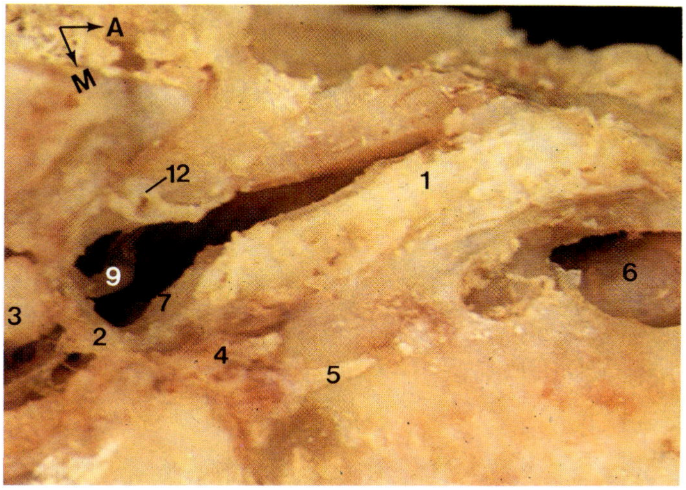

1 Tensor tympani muscle
2 Tensor tympani tendon
3 Head of malleus
4 Geniculate ganglion
5 Greater superficial petrosal nerve
6 Internal carotid artery
7 Edge of bony semicanal for tensor tympani muscle
8 Bony tympanic annulus
9 Umbo of malleus
10 Superior malleolar ligament
11 Incudo-stapedial joint
12 Chorda tympani
13 Plicae of mucosa of the mastoid cavity

46

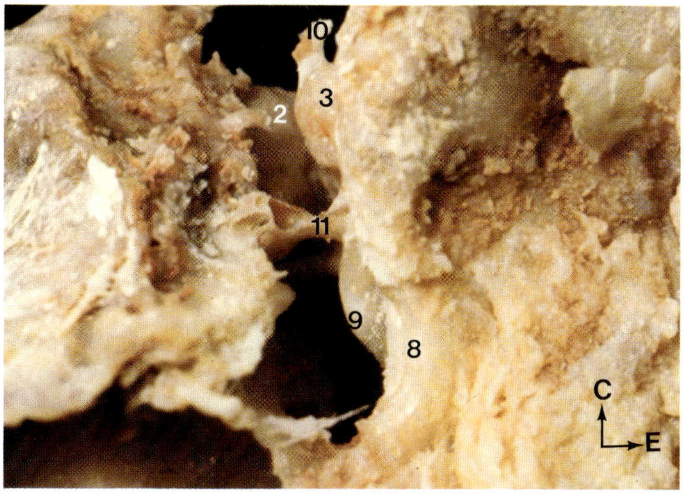

46 Anterior view of tympanic cavity (bony Eustachian tube removed)

47

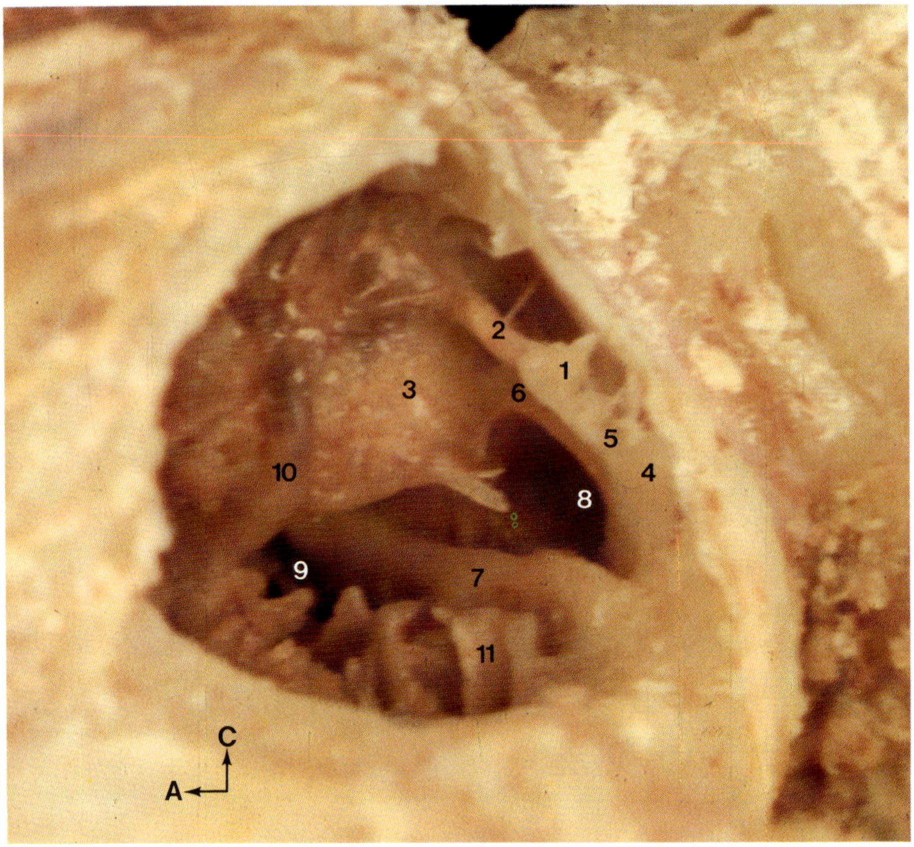

47 Posterior view of the left hypotympanum, (tympanic membrane, malleus and incus removed)

48

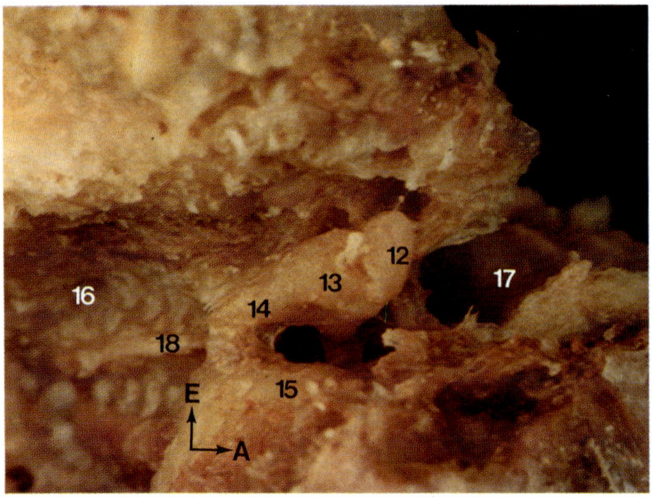

48 Postero-superior view of tympanic cavity (tegmen removed)

1 Head of stapes
2 Anterior crus of stapes
3 Promontory
4 Pyramid
5 Stapedial tendon
6 Ponticulus
7 Subiculum
8 Tympanic sinus
9 Round window fossa
10 Tympanic branch (Jacobson's) of the glossopharyngeal nerve
11 Hypotympanic air cells
12 Head of malleus
13 Body of incus
14 Short process of incus
15 Lateral semicircular canal
16 Mastoid cavity
17 Middle ear cavity
18 Chorda tympani

49 & 50 Posterior view of left tympanic cavity (tegmen removed)

49

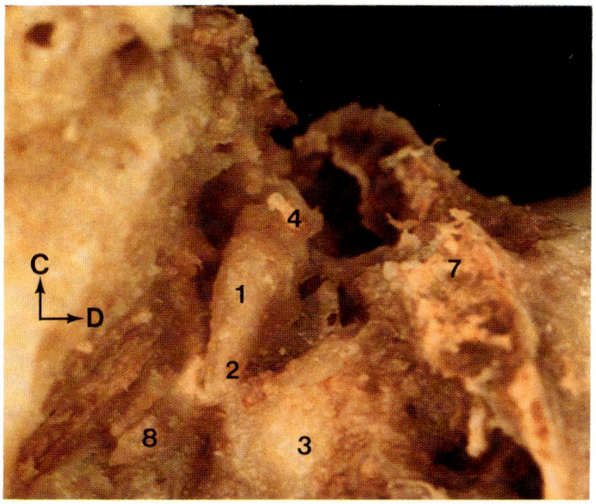

50

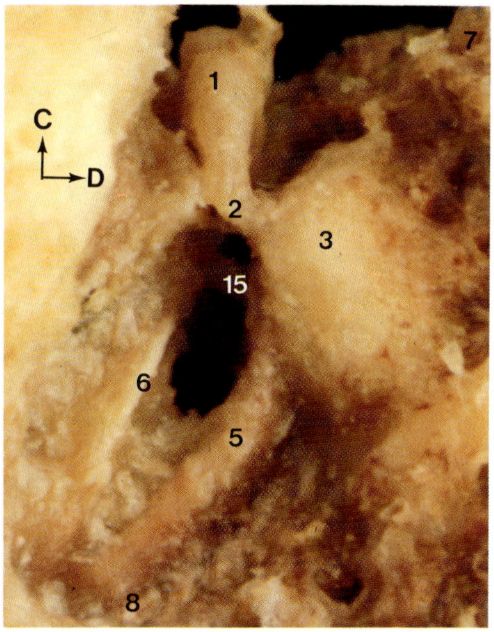

1 Body of incus
2 Short process of incus
3 Lateral semicircular canal
4 Head of malleus
5 Facial nerve
6 Chorda tympani
7 Tegmen tympani (cut edge)
8 Mastoid cavity
9 Stapes
10 Cut edge of posterior wall of external auditory meatus
11 Semicanal of tensor tympani muscle
12 Basal turn of cochlea
13 Round window membrane
14 Hypotympanum
15 Incudo-stapedial joint

Note: The short process of the incus is of great surgical importance for pin-pointing the facial nerve.

51 Posterior view of left hypotympanum (tympanic membrane, malleus, incus and lower promontory removed)

51

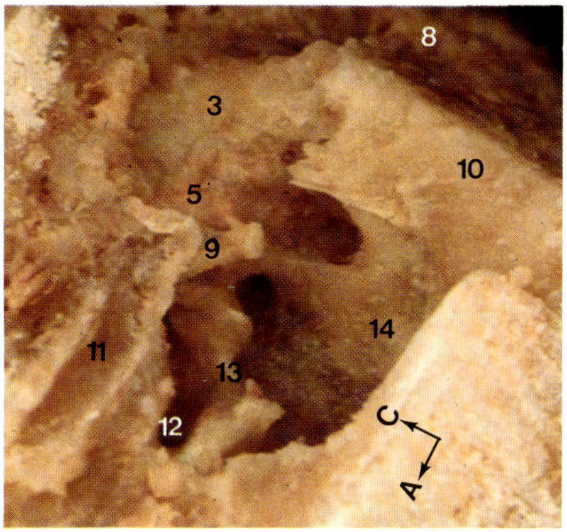

52

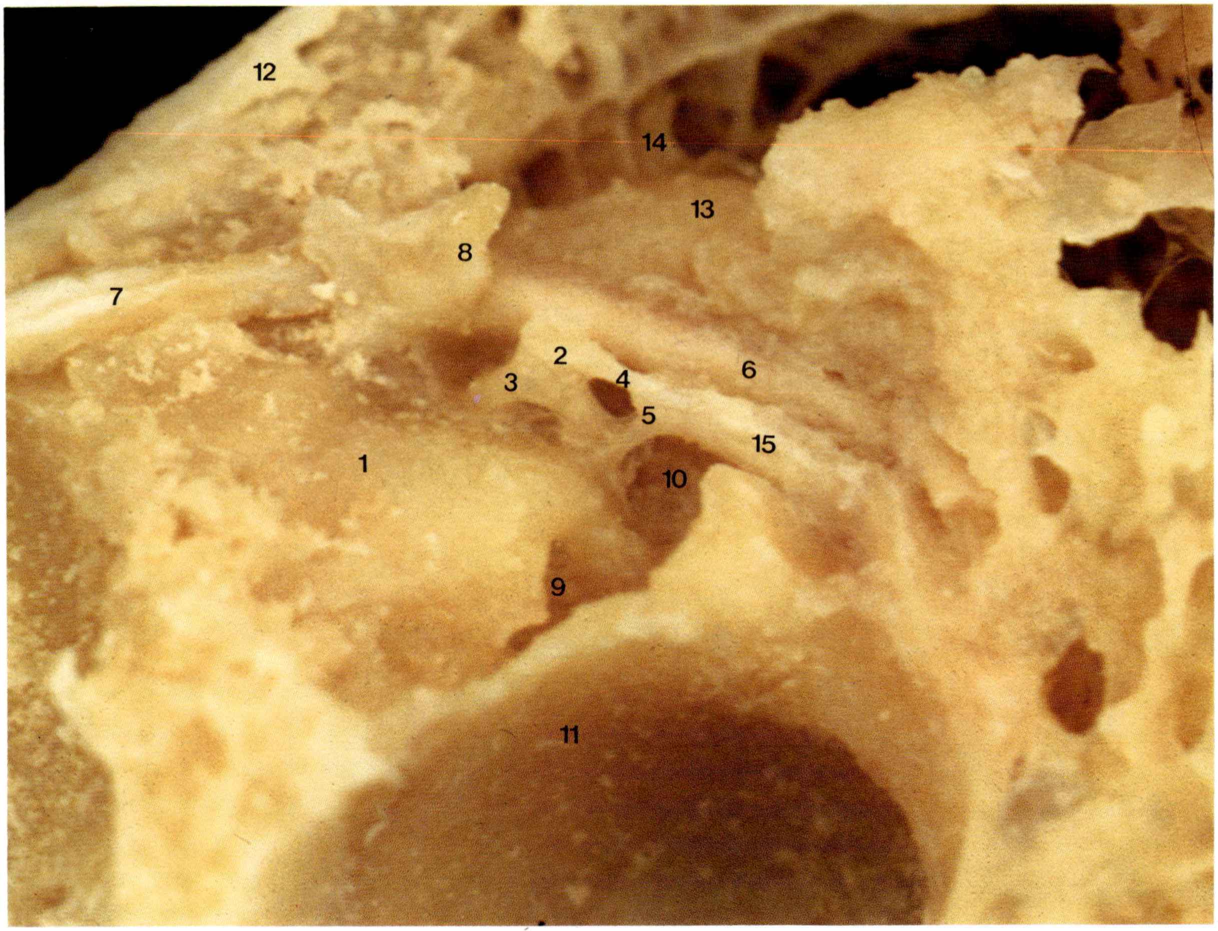

52 Lateral view of medial wall of left tympanic cavity

1 Promontory
2 Head of stapes
3 Anterior crus of stapes
4 Stapedius tendon
5 Pyramid
6 Facial nerve
7 Tensor tympani tendon
8 Cochleariform process
9 Round window fossa
10 Tympanic sinus
11 Jugular fossa
12 Tegmen tympani
13 Lateral semicircular canal
14 Mastoid antrum
15 Stapedius muscle

Note: The facial nerve may be more lateral than the lateral semicircular canal.

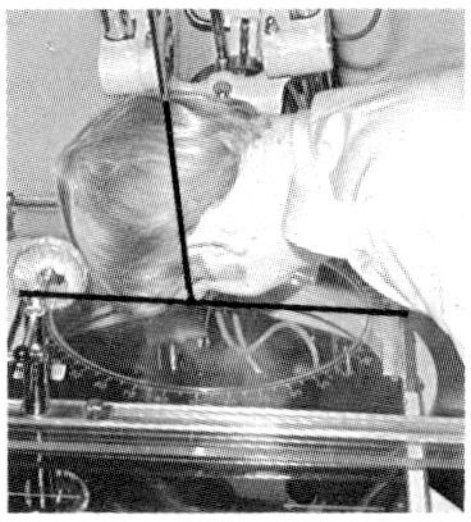

Guillen's radiographic position

53

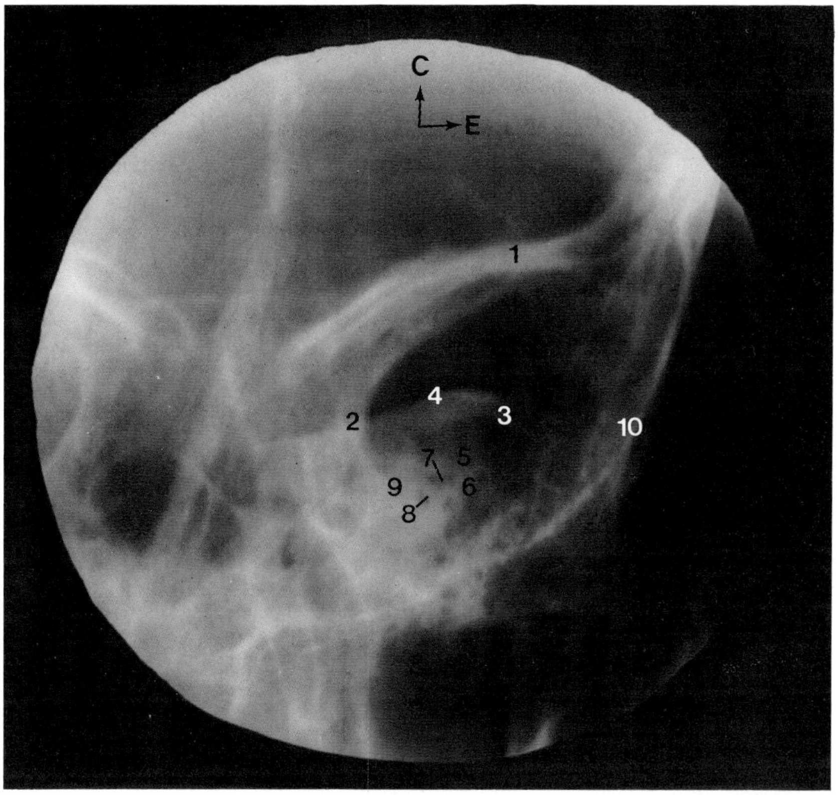

53 Left transorbital (Guillen's) radiograph

54

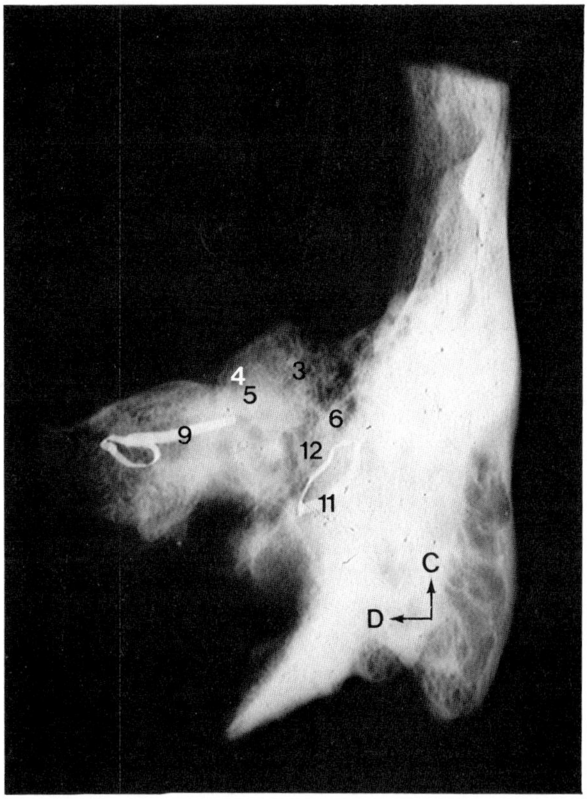

54 Guillen's radiograph of dry temporal bone

1 Supra-orbital margin
2 Medial orbital margin
3 Tegmen tympani
4 Arcuate eminence
5 Superior semicircular canal
6 Ossicles
7 Lateral semicircular canal
8 Facial nerve canal
9 Internal auditory canal
10 Lateral orbital margin
11 Tympanic ring
12 Middle ear

55

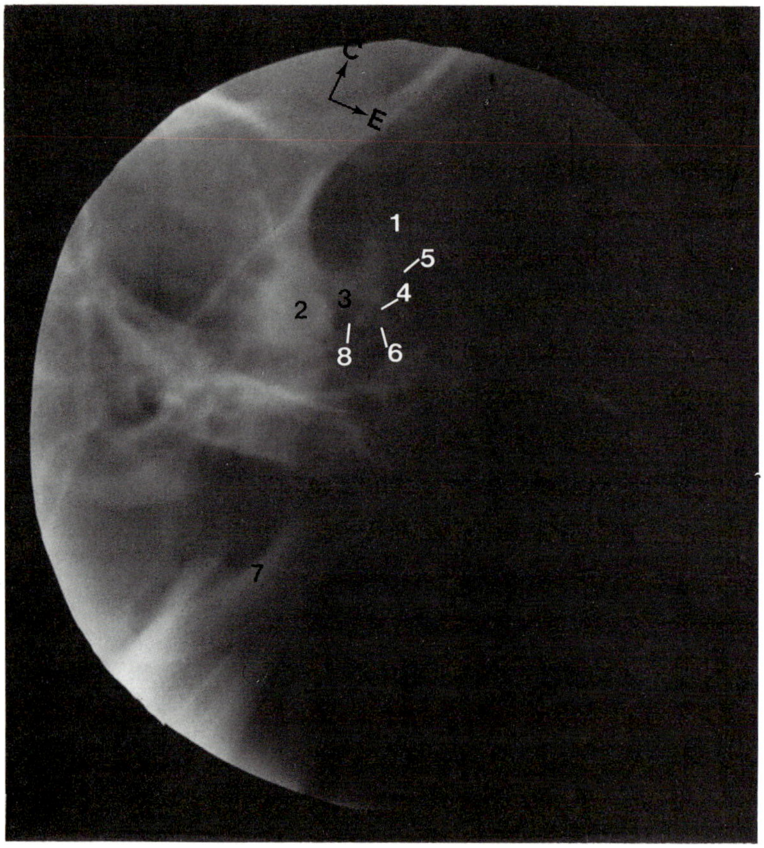

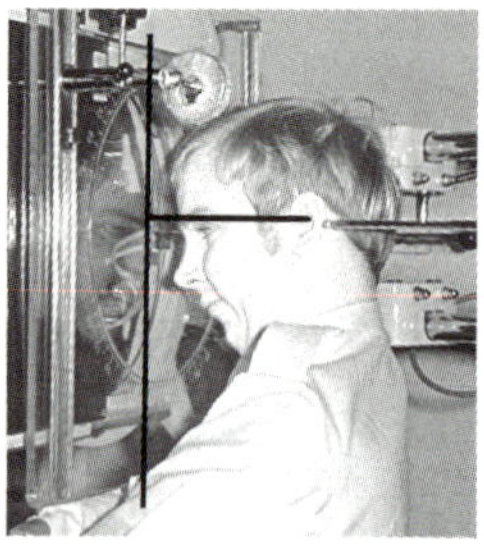

Chaussée III radiographic position

55 Left Chaussée III radiograph

56

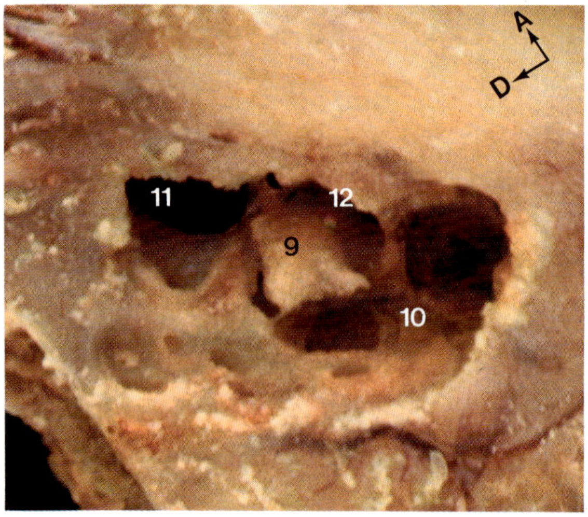

56 Superior view of mastoid cavity

1 Arcuate eminence
2 Cochlea
3 Vestibule
4 Lateral semicircular canal
5 Superior semicircular canal
6 Facial nerve canal
7 Mandible
8 Oval window
9 Incus
10 Plicae of mucous membrane in the mastoid cavity
11 Middle ear cavity
12 Edges of the cut tegmen

57 Anterior wall of left mastoid cavity (tegmen removed)

1 Cut edges of tegmen
2 Body of incus
3 Fossa incudis
4 Lateral semicircular canal
5 Facial nerve
6 Chorda tympani
7 Incudo-stapedial joint
8 Superior ligament
9 Lateral sinus plate
10 Posterior wall of the external auditory canal
11 External auditory canal
12 Digastric ridge
13 Stapes
14 Sterno-mastoid muscle
15 Tegmen
16 Posterior fossa cortex
17 Endolymphatic sac
18 Antrum
19 Sino-dural angle

Note: a) A good view of the middle ear is obtained between the chorda tympani and facial nerve.
b) The vertical portion of the facial nerve may be divided into two or three separate branches.

57

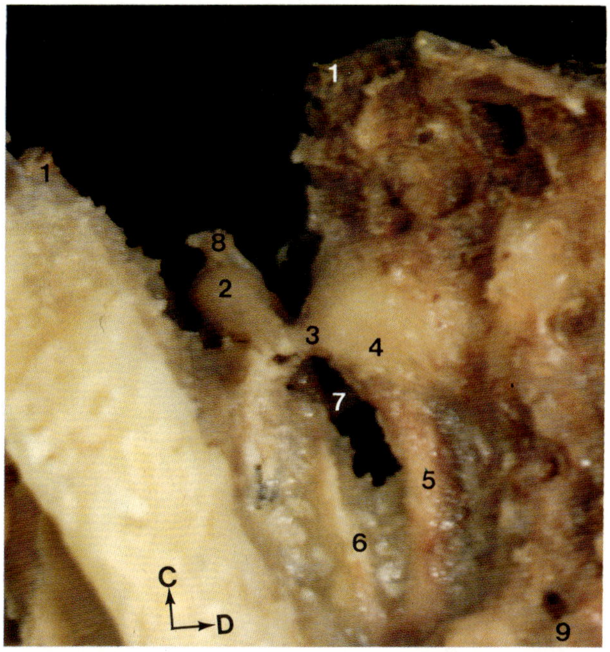

58

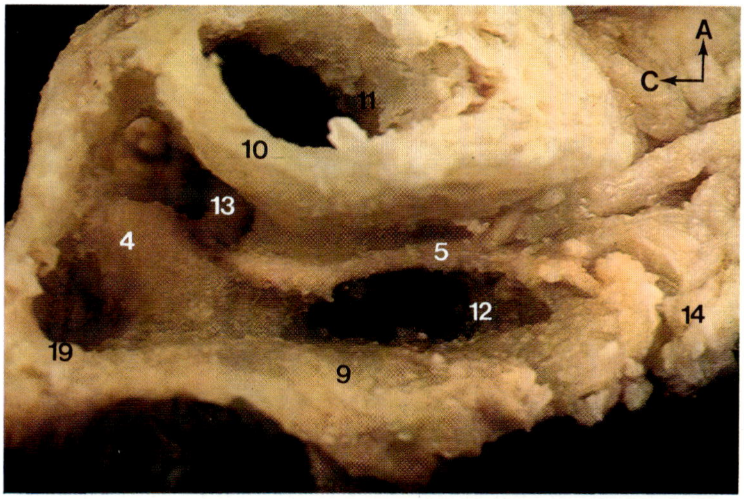

58 Mastoid cavity with intact wall technique

59

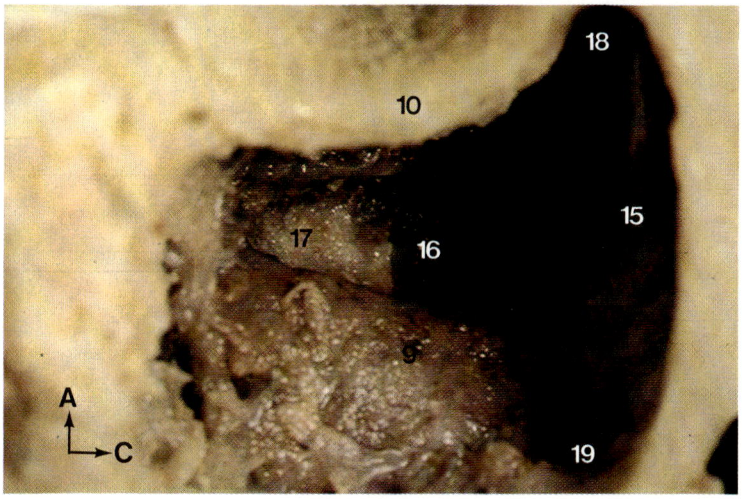

59 Mastoid cavity to show endolymphatic sac situation

60

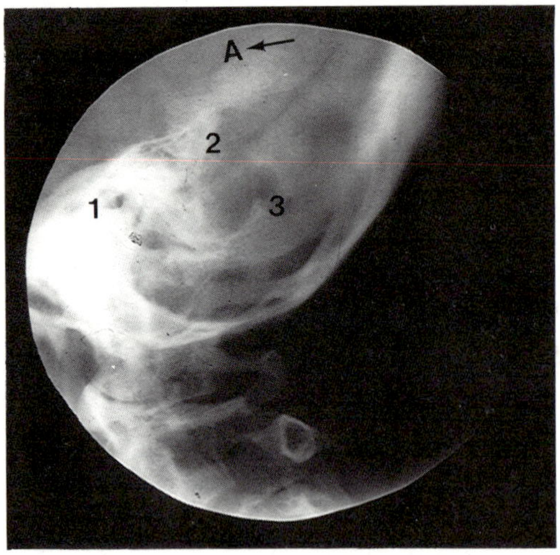

60 Lateral radiograph of mastoid

61

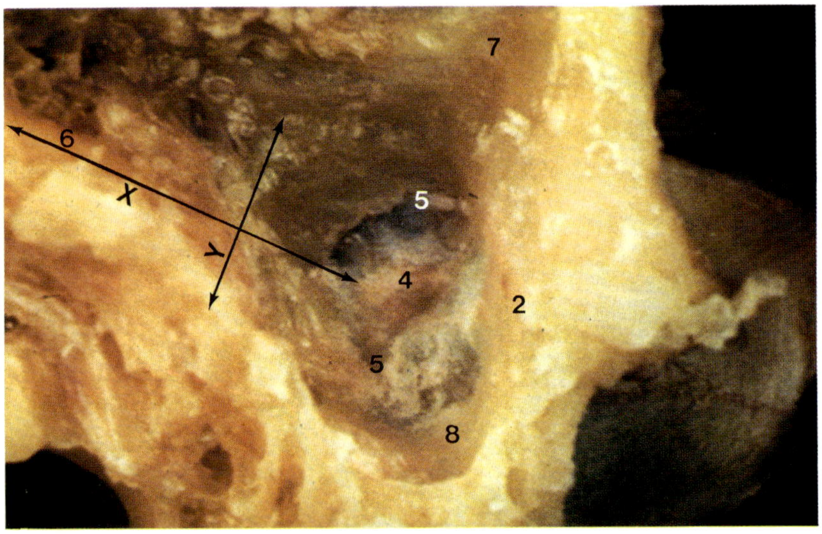

61 Left mastoid cavity to demonstrate the endolymphatic sac

1 Petrous temporal bone
2 Lateral sinus with anterior plate
3 Mastoid emissary vein
4 Endolymphatic sac
5 Dura of posterior fossa superiorly and inferiorly exposed
6 Lateral semicircular canal
7 Sino-dural angle
8 Digastric ridge

Note: The lateral semicircular canal axis (X) and the posterior semicircular canal axis (Y) are useful aids in finding the endolymphtic sac. The lateral sinus may be exposed down to the posterior fossa dura which shows blue around a white endolymphatic sac.

62

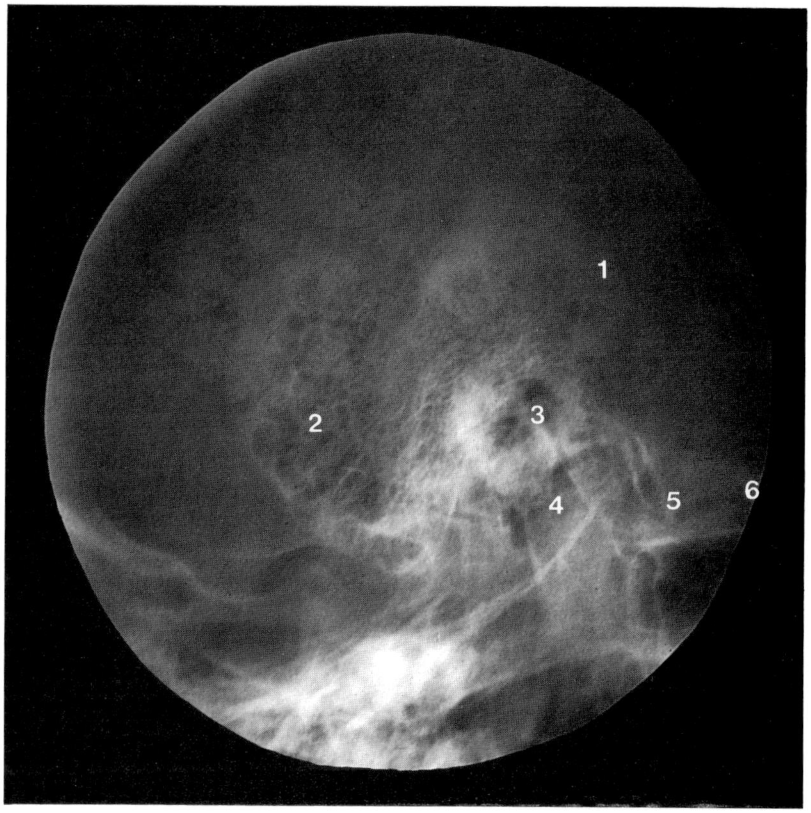

62 Lateral radiograph

1 Pinna
2 Very cellular mastoid
3 Superimposed internal and external auditory canals
4 Mandibular condyle
5 Articular eminence
6 Zygomatic arch

63

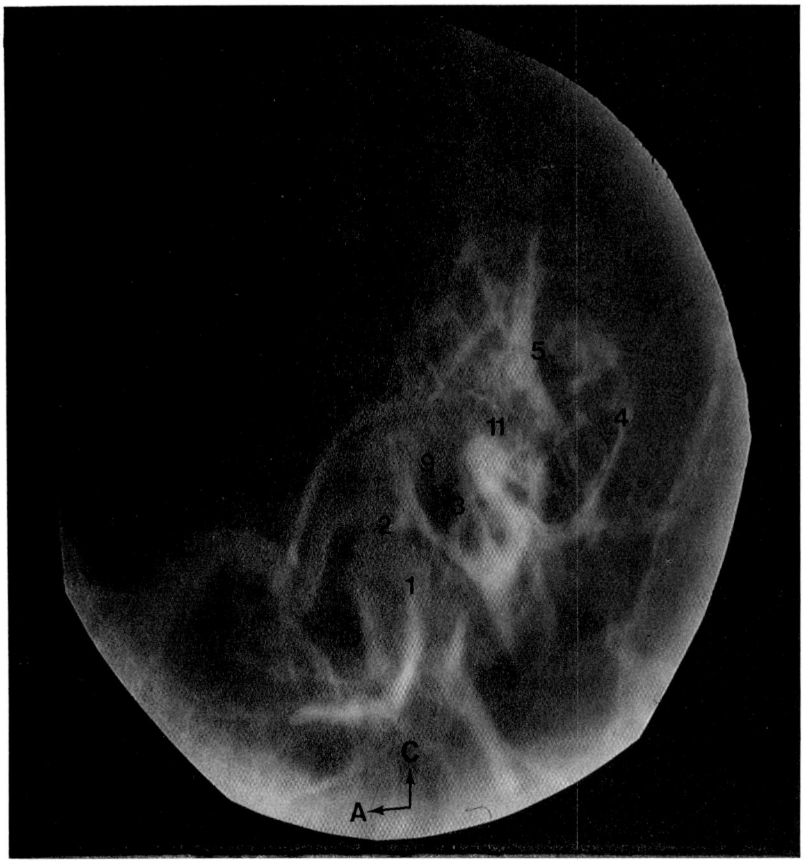

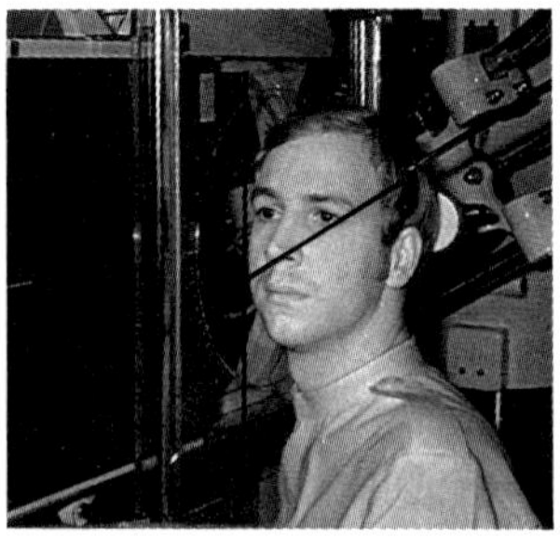

Schüller's position (lateral oblique)

63 Lateral (Owen's position) radiograph (modified Mayer's)

64

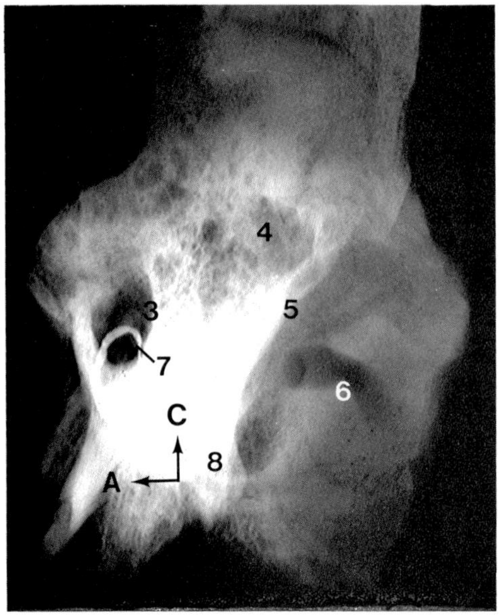

64 Owen's position with a dry bone

1 Condyle of mandible
2 Mandibular fossa
3 Middle ear through the external auditory canal
4 Mastoid cells
5 Lateral sinus and plate
6 Mastoid emissary vein
7 Tympanic ring
8 Internal auditory meatus
9 Ossicles
10 Tempero-mandibular joint
11 Aditus

Note: The lateral positions are variations of beam angle to prevent superimposition of bilateral structures.

The Owen's position gives the view most recognisable to the surgeon with the ossicles in the normal position.

65 Lateral (Mayer's position) radiograph

65

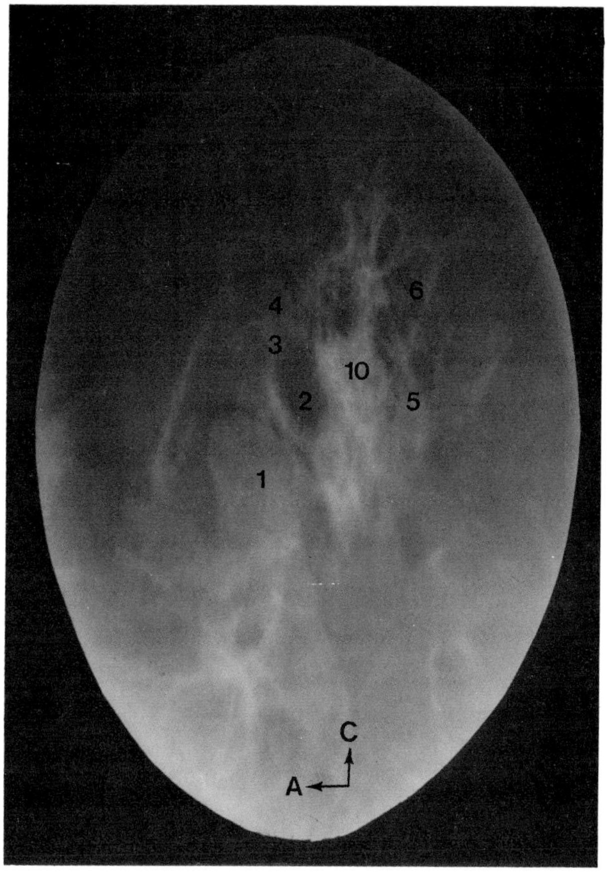

1 Condyle of mandible
2 Middle ear through the external auditory canal
3 Ossicles in attic
4 Aditus
5 Lateral sinus and plate
6 Mastoid cells
7 Mastoid emissary vein
8 Internal auditory meatus
9 Tympanic ring
10 Cochlear area

66

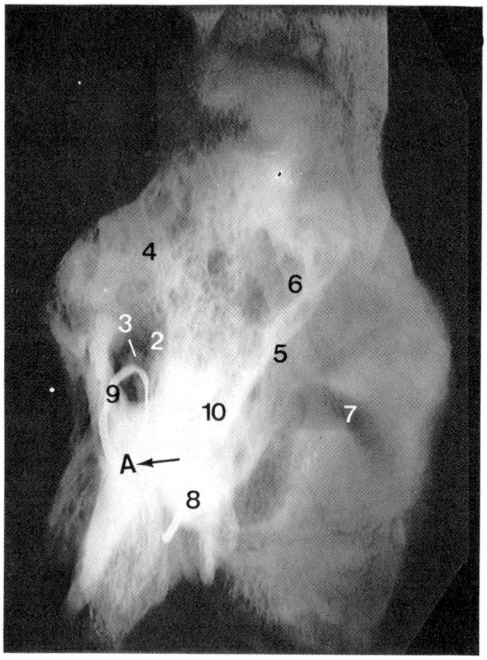

66 Mayer's position with dry bone

67

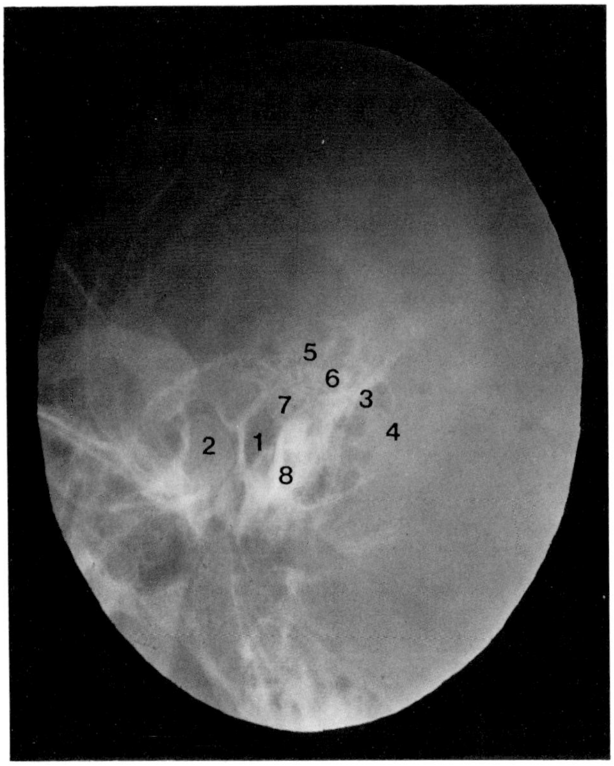

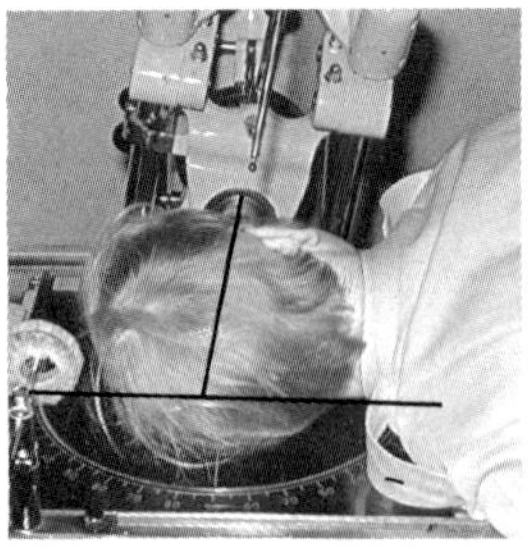

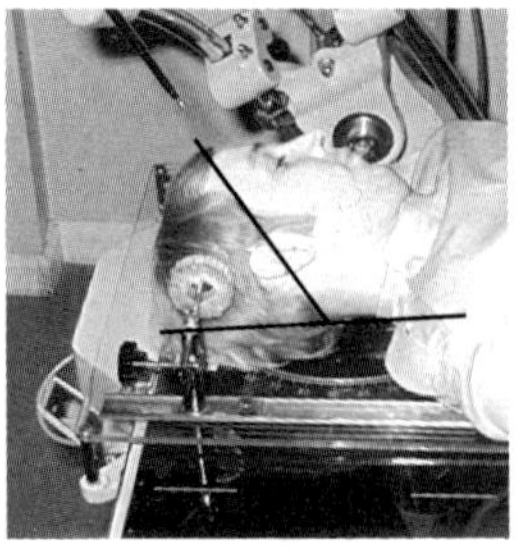

Stockholm (lateral oblique views) positions 'B' and 'C'

67 Stockholm 'B' 30°-35° lateral oblique radiograph

68

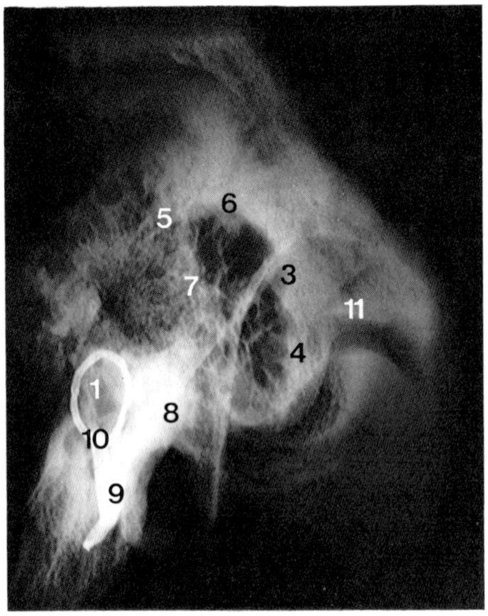

68 Stockholm 'B' radiograph of dry bone

1 External auditory canal overlying the middle ear and internal auditory canal
2 Condyle of mandible
3 Lateral sinus plate
4 Petro-sinus cells (marginal)
5 Squamous cells
6 Upper margin of petrous bone
7 Antrum and aditus
8 Labyrinth
9 Internal auditory canal
10 Tympanic ring
11 Mastoid emissary vein

69 Stockholm 'C' radiograph (very similar to Stenver's)

69

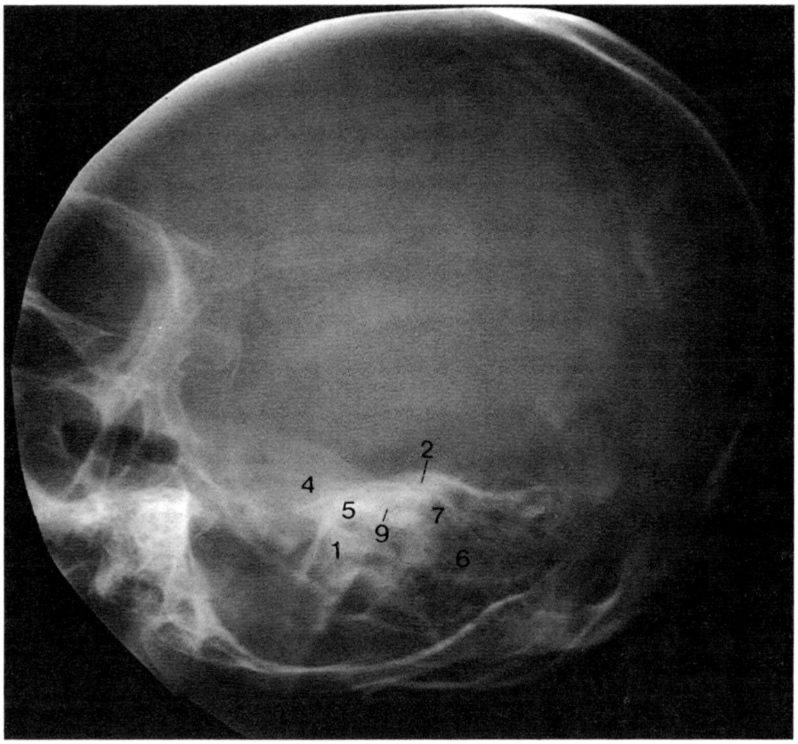

1 Condyle of mandible
2 Arcuate eminence
3 Superior semicircular canal
4 Petrous apex
5 Internal auditory canal
6 Mastoid cells
7 Antral cells
8 Tympanic ring
9 Vestibule

70

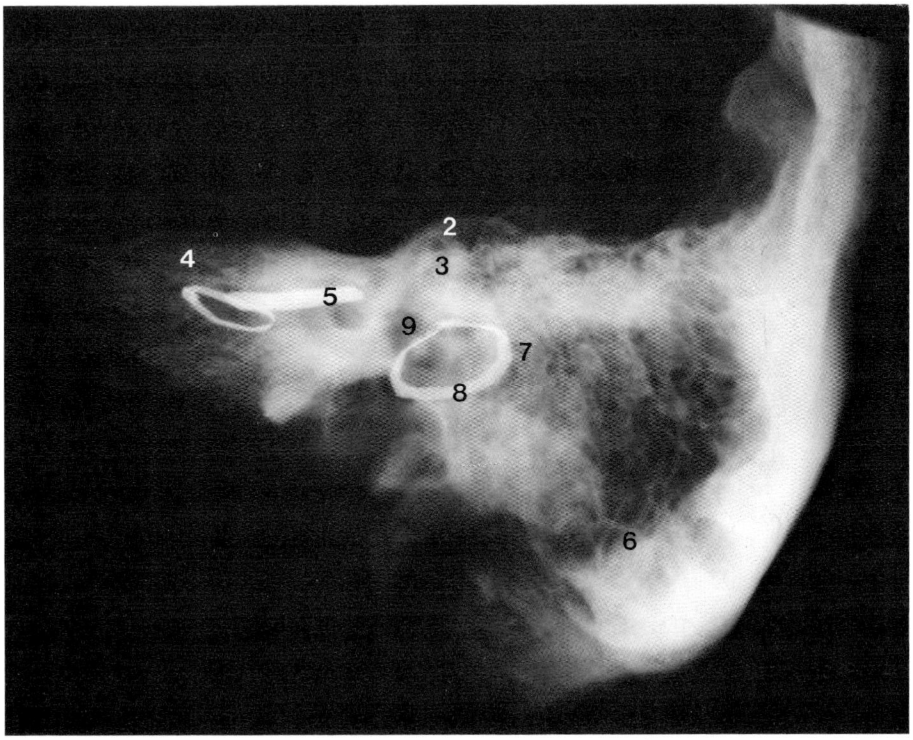

70 Stockholm 'C' radiograph of dry bone

71

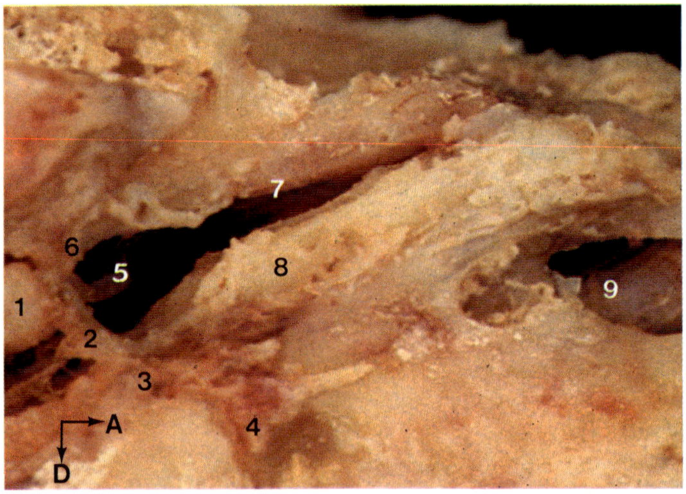

71 Superior view of eustachian tube (tegmen removed)

72

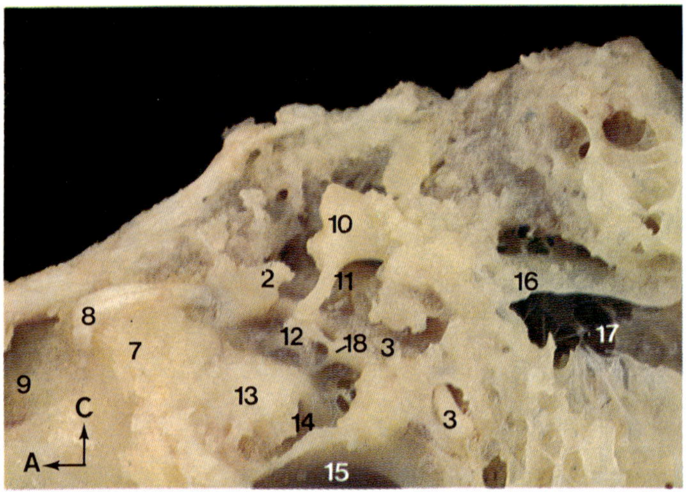

72 Lateral view of the medial wall of a left middle ear

1 Head of malleus
2 Tendon of tensor tympani muscle
3 Facial nerve
4 Geniculate ganglion area
5 Umbo (medial surface)
6 Chorda tympani (in petrotympanic fissure)
7 Bony eustachian tube (roof removed)
8 Tensor tympani muscle
9 Carotid canal
10 Body of incus
11 Lateral semicircular canal
12 Stapes
13 Promontory
14 Round window fossa
15 Jugular fossa
16 Körner's septum
17 Mastoid cavity cells
18 Pyramid and stapedius tendon

73

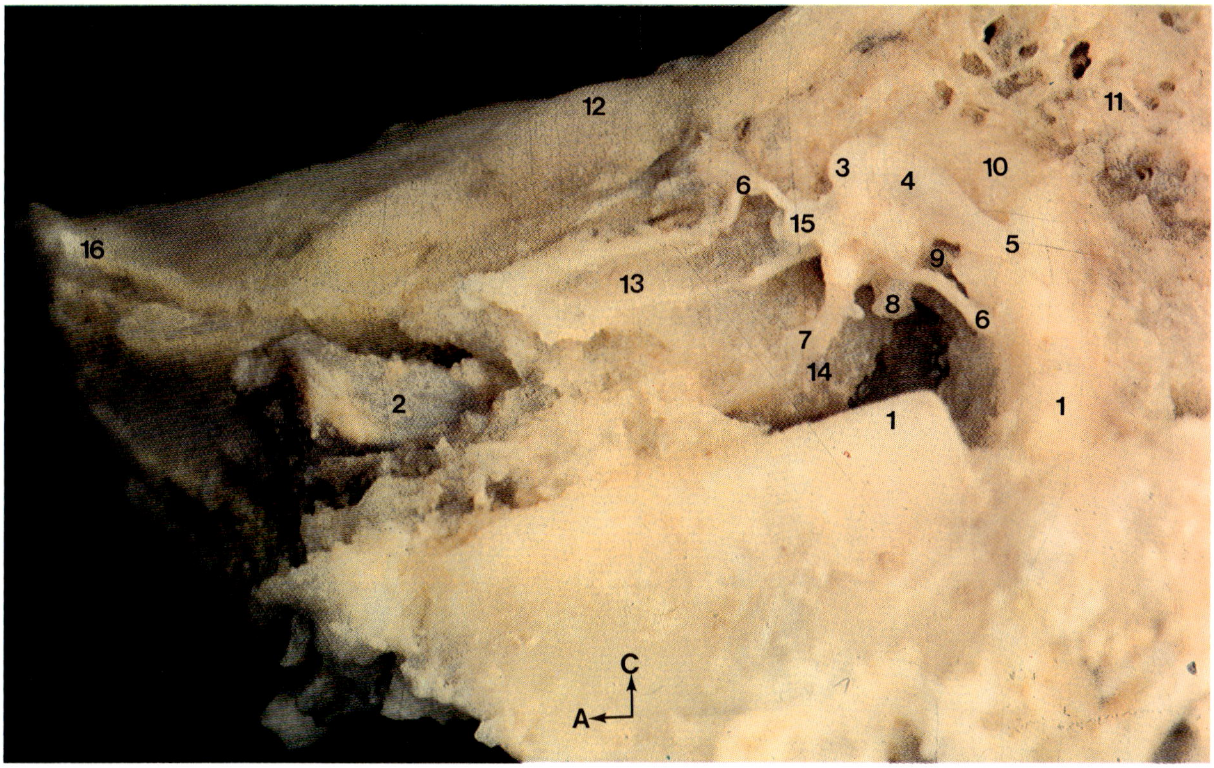

73 Lateral view of the medial wall of a left middle ear

1 Cut edges of the external auditory canal
2 Carotid artery in the canal
3 Malleus head
4 Incus body
5 Fossa incudis
6 Chorda tympani
7 Umbo (tympanic membrane removed)
8 Lentiform process
9 Facial nerve
10 Lateral semicircular canal
11 Mastoid cells
12 Tegmen (removed)
13 Semicanal for the tensor tympani muscle
14 Promontory
15 Cochleariform process
16 Petrous tip

74

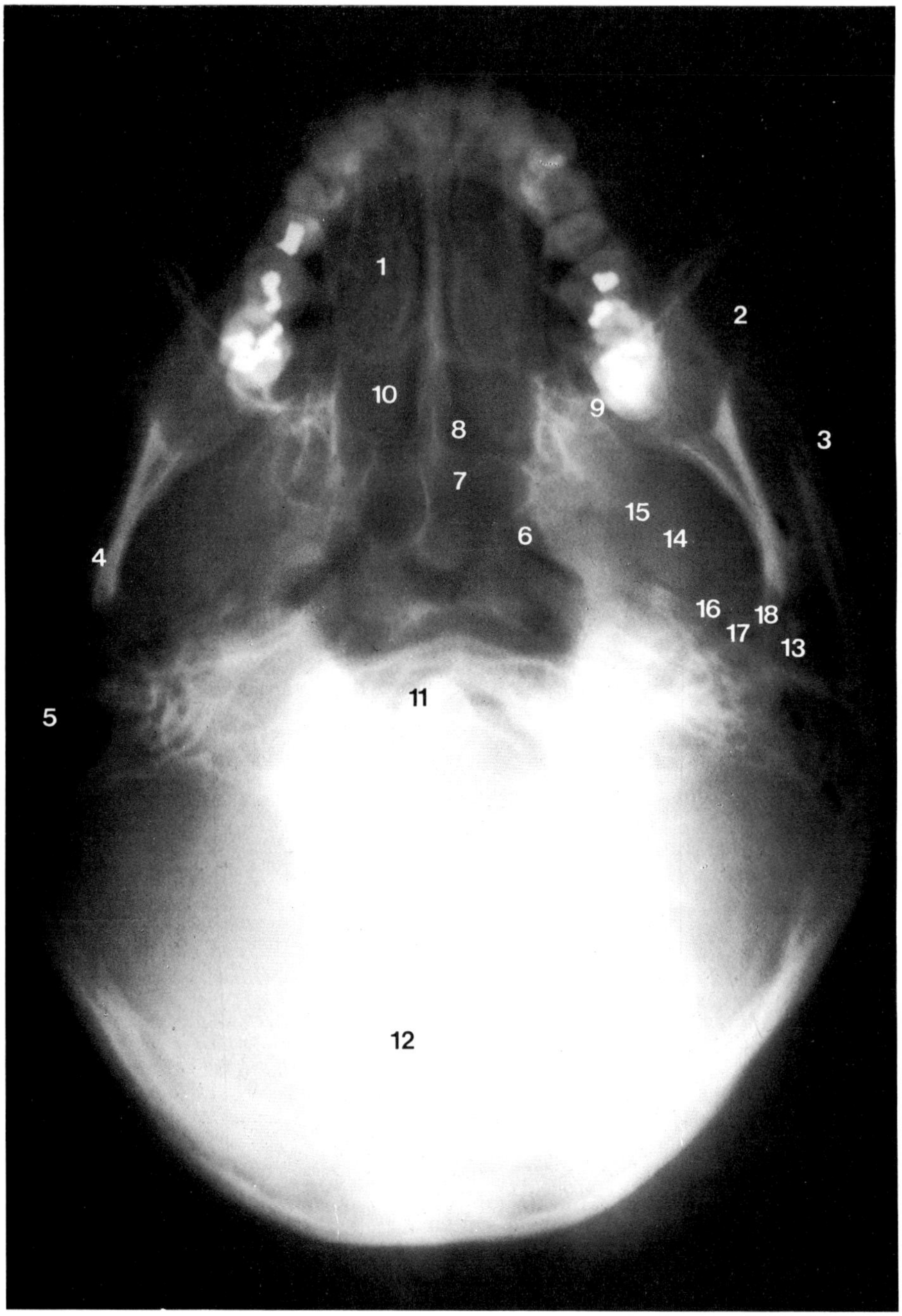

74 Submento-vertical radiograph

1 Palatine process of the maxilla
2 Lateral wall of the maxilla
3 Zygomatic arch
4 Mandibular fossa
5 Mastoid process
6 Petrous temporal apex
7 Sphenoid body
8 Vomer
9 Lateral pterygoid plate
10 Posterior nares
11 Foramen magnum
12 Occipital bone
13 External auditory meatus
14 Foramen spinosum
15 Foramen ovale
16 Bony eustachian tube
17 Middle ear cavity
18 Ossicles (malleus and incus superimposed)

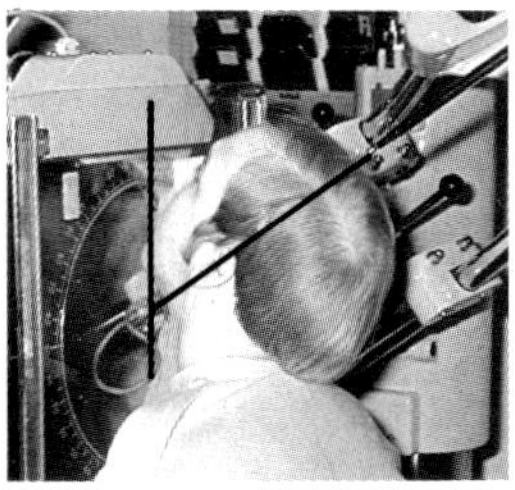

Occipito-mental radiographic position

75

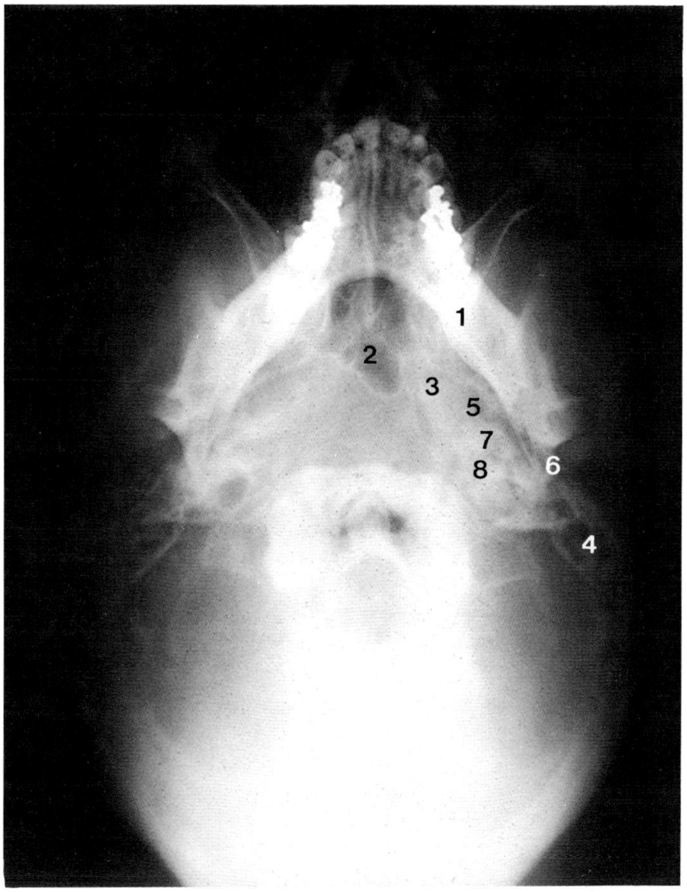

75 Occipito-mental radiograph

1 Mandible
2 Sphenoid sinus
3 Petrous tip
4 Mastoid cells
5 Eustachian tube
6 External auditory canal
7 Cochlea
8 Internal auditory canal
9 Tympanic ring

76

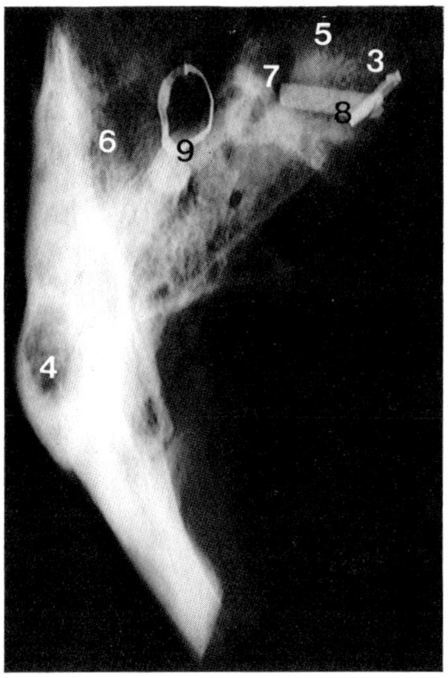

76 Occipito-mental radiograph of a dry bone

77

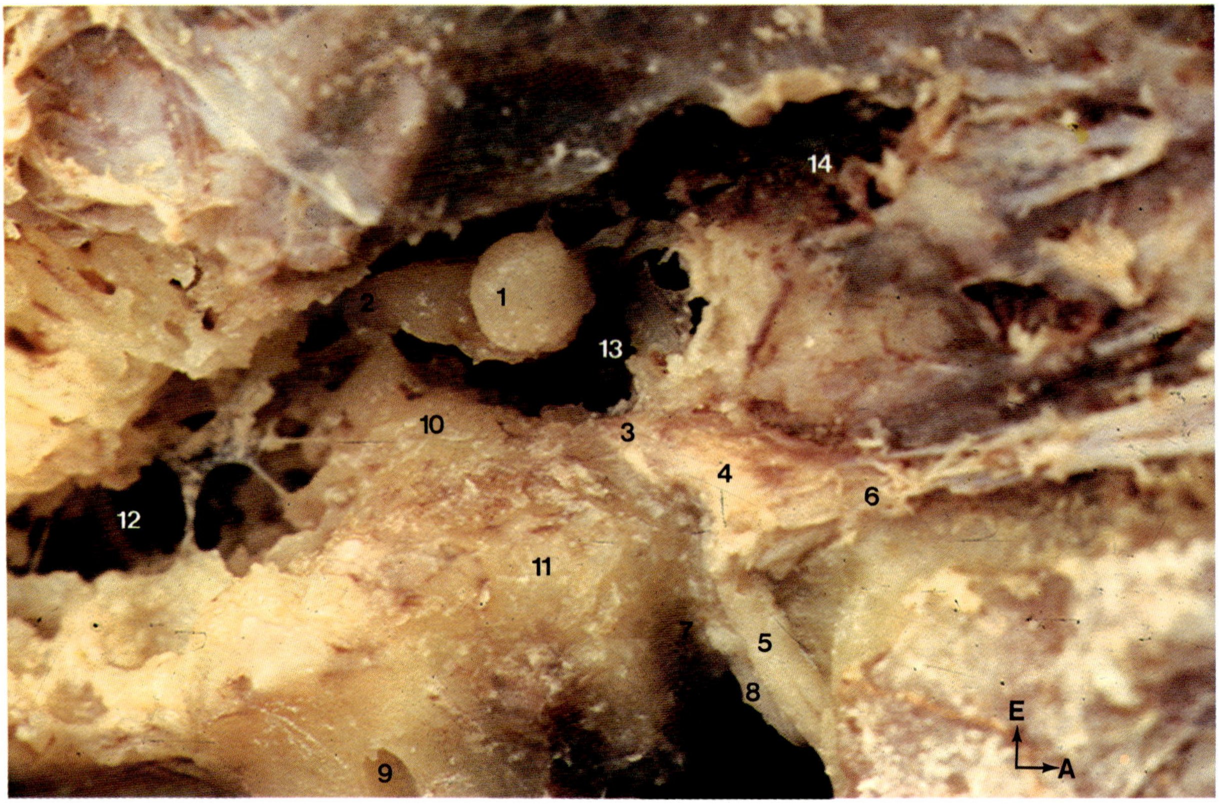

77 Superior view of the left middle ear with the tegmen removed

1 Head of malleus
2 Short process of incus
3 Facial nerve
4 Geniculate ganglion of facial nerve
5 Facial nerve in the internal auditory canal
6 Greater superficial petrosal nerve
7 Fundus of the internal auditory canal
8 Vestibular nerve (superior part)
9 Superior semicircular canal
10 Area of lateral semicircular canal
11 Area of cochlea
12 Mastoid cavity with mucosal webs
13 Tensor tympani tendon
14 Opening of eustachian tube

78

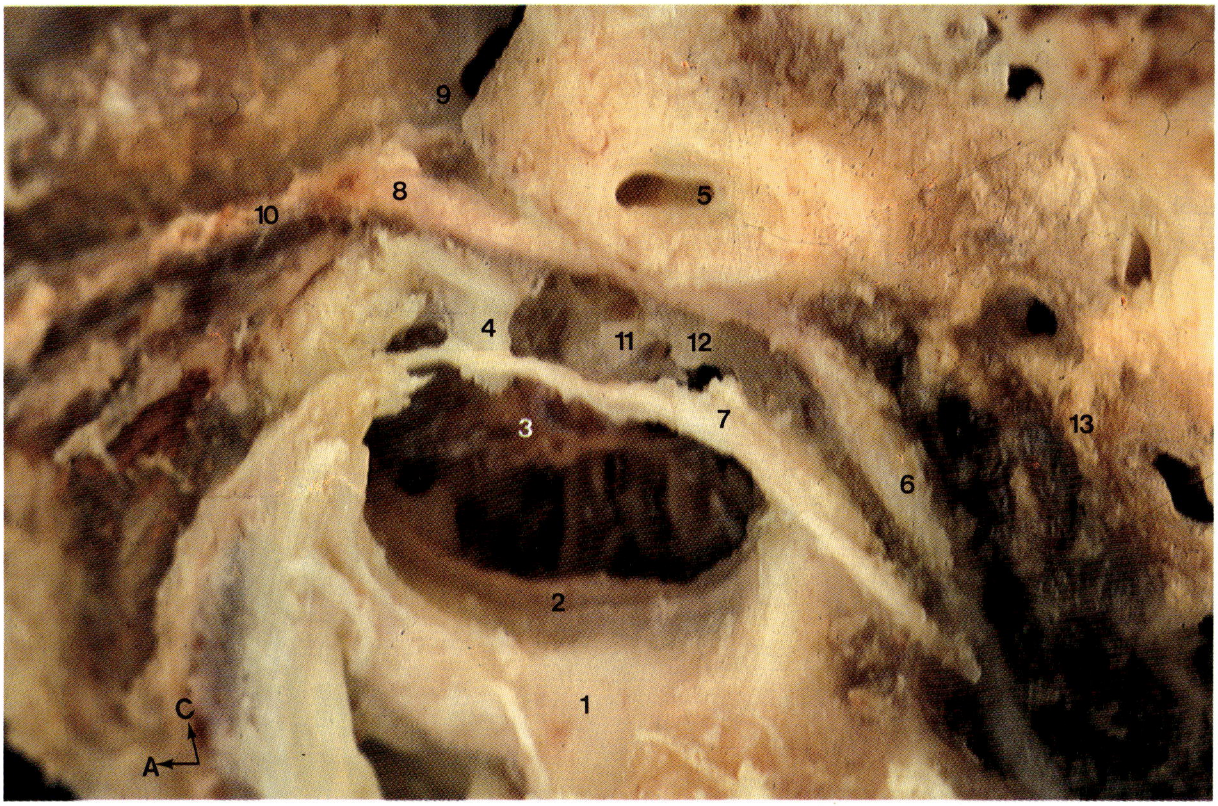

78 Supero-lateral view of tegmen area after removal of tympanic membrane and ossicles

1 External auditory canal
2 Groove for tympanic ring
3 Promontory
4 Cochleariform process
5 Lateral semicircular canal
6 Facial nerve (vertical portion)
7 Chorda tympani
8 Geniculate ganglion of facial nerve
9 Fundus of the internal auditory canal
10 Greater superficial petrosal nerve
11 Head of stapes
12 Pyramid
13 Mastoid cavity

79

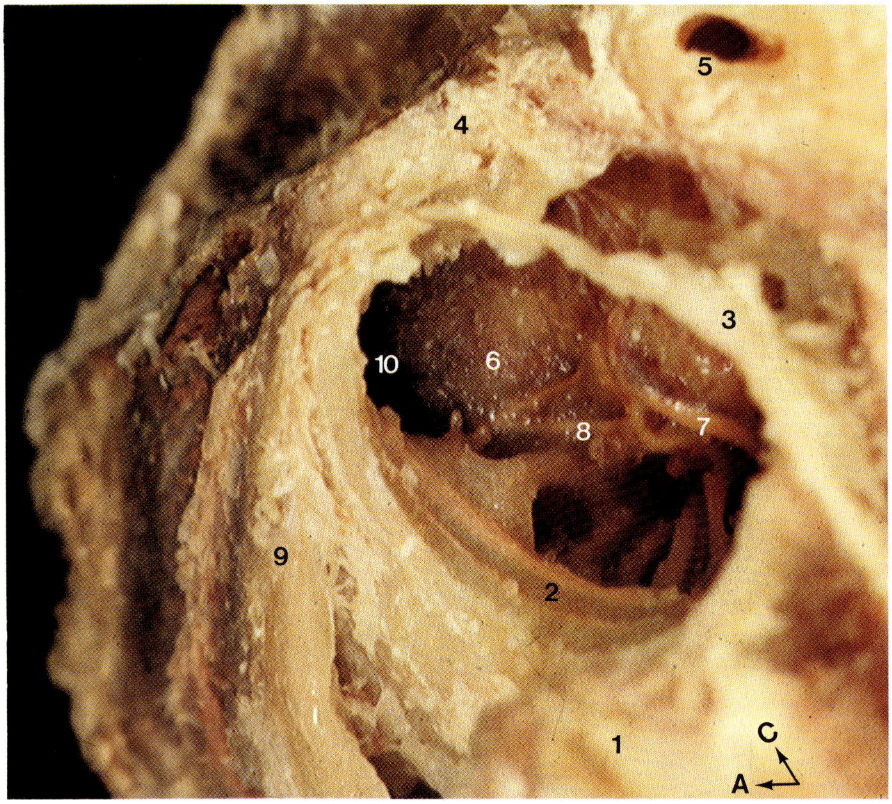

79 Lateral view of the left chorda tympani and anterior hypotympanum after removal of the tympanic membrane and ossicles

1 External auditory meatus
2 Groove for tympanic ring
3 Chorda tympani
4 Facial nerve
5 Lateral semicircular canal
6 Anterior promontory
7 Jacobson's nerve (IX)
8 Hypotympanic branch of Jacobsen's nerve
9 Temperomandibular joint tissues
10 Eustachian tube opening

Note: Jacobson's nerve arises from the IXth cranial nerve in the jugular foramen and crosses the promontory to the geniculate ganglion. It then becomes the lesser superficial petrosal nerve carrying parasympathetic fibres to the parotid gland.

80 A supero-lateral view of the anterior part of the chorda tympani

80

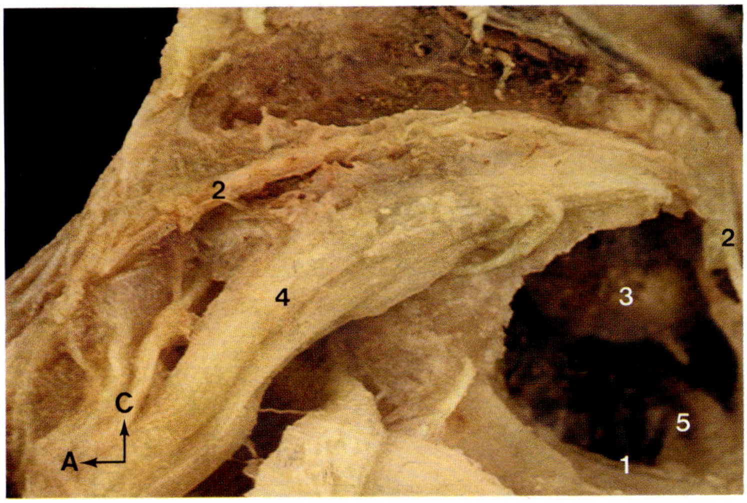

81

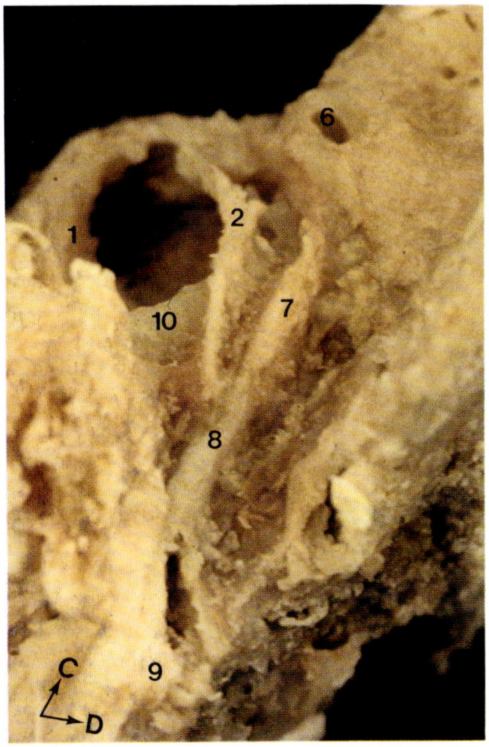

1 Groove for tympanic ring
2 Chorda tympani in the petrotympanic fissure
3 Promontory
4 Temperomandibular joint tissues
5 Hypotympanum
6 Lateral semicircular canal
7 Facial nerve (vertical portion)
8 Junction of chorda tympani and facial nerve
9 Deep part of the mastoid cavity
10 Posterior wall of the external auditory canal

81 Posterior view of the vertical position of the facial nerve and chorda tympani

82

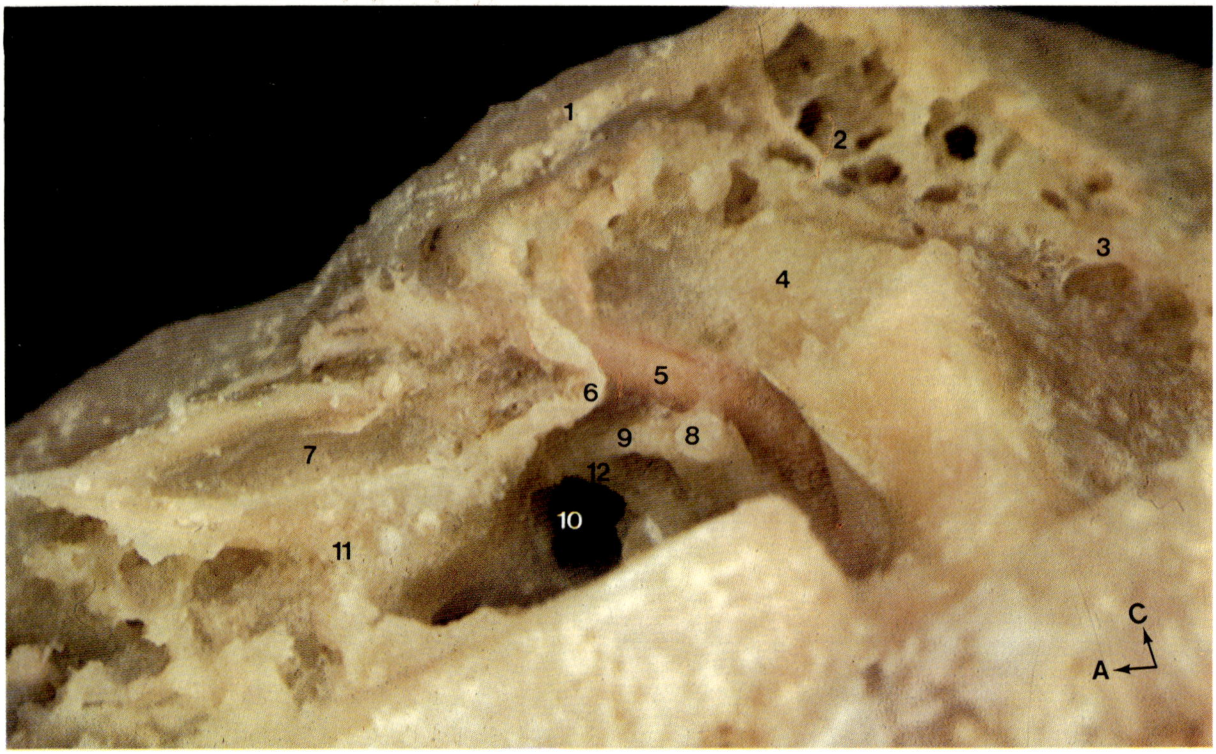

82 Lateral view of the medial wall of the left middle ear cavity

1 Tegmen tympani
2 Mastoid cells in the aditus
3 Antrum
4 Lateral semicircular canal
5 Facial nerve
6 Cochleariform process with tendon removed
7 Semicanal for tensor tympani muscle
8 Head of the stapes
10 Tympanic sinus
11 Eustachian tube opening
12 Ponticulus

83

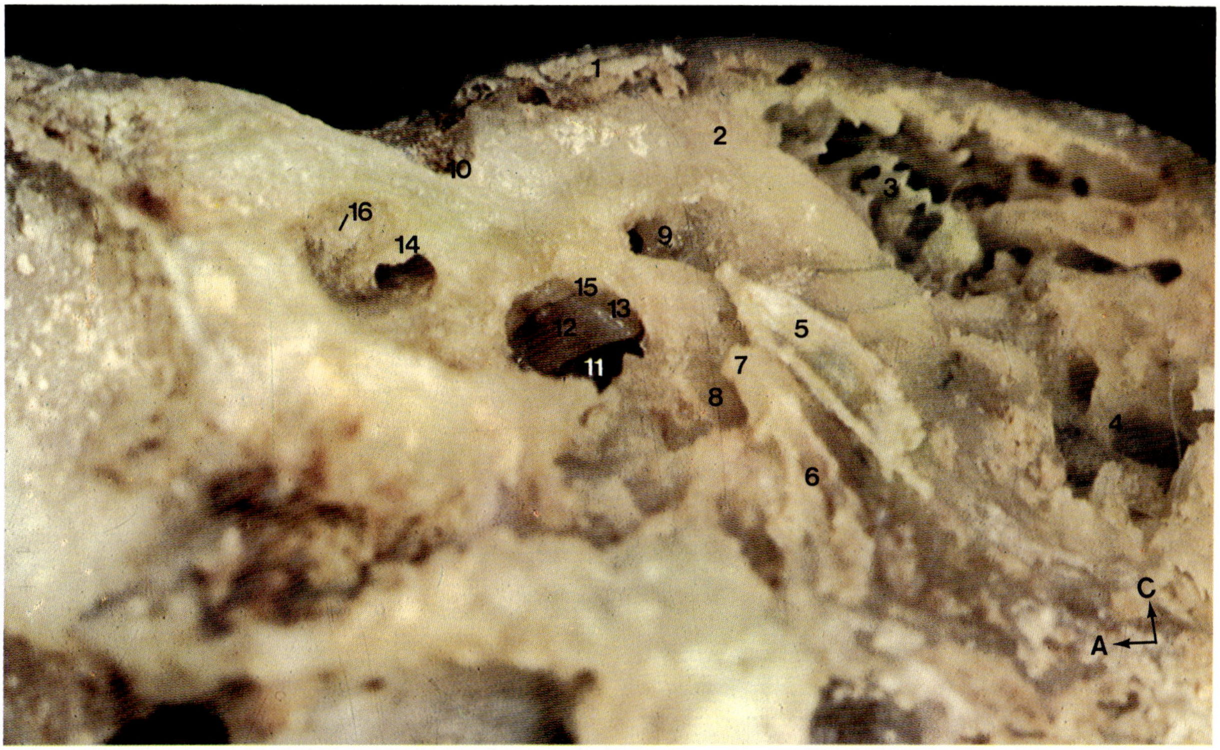

83 Lateral view of the medial wall of the left middle ear and cochlea

1 Tegmen tympani
2 Aditus
3 Antral cells
4 Mastoid cavity
5 Facial nerve (removed) sheath
6 Stapedius muscle remnants
7 Tip of pyramid
8 Tympanic sinus
9 Lateral semicircular canal
10 Groove for facial nerve at the geniculate ganglion
11 Vestibule
12 Saccule
13 Utricle
14 Osseous spiral ligament of the cochlea
15 Edge of enlarged oval window
16 Cochlea

84

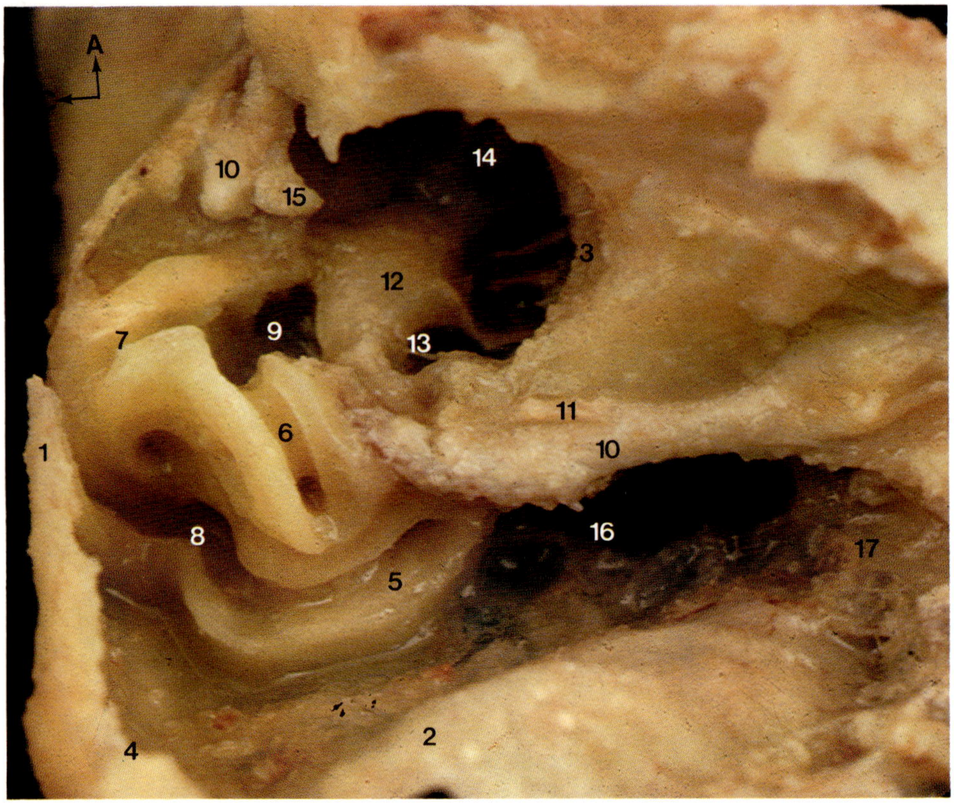

84 Lateral view of a right osseous labyrinth

1 Tegmen tympani
2 Lateral sinus plate
3 Groove for tympanic ring
4 Sino-dural angle
5 Posterior semicircular canal
6 Lateral semicircular canal
7 Superior semicircular canal (arcuate eminence)
8 Crus commune
9 Vestibule viewed through enlarged oval window
10 Facial nerve (cut at the oval window)
11 Chorda tympani (cut)
12 Promontory
13 Round window fossa
14 Hypotympanic cells leading towards Eustachian opening
15 Cochleariform process
16 Retro-facial cells
17 Digastric ridge in mastoid tip

85

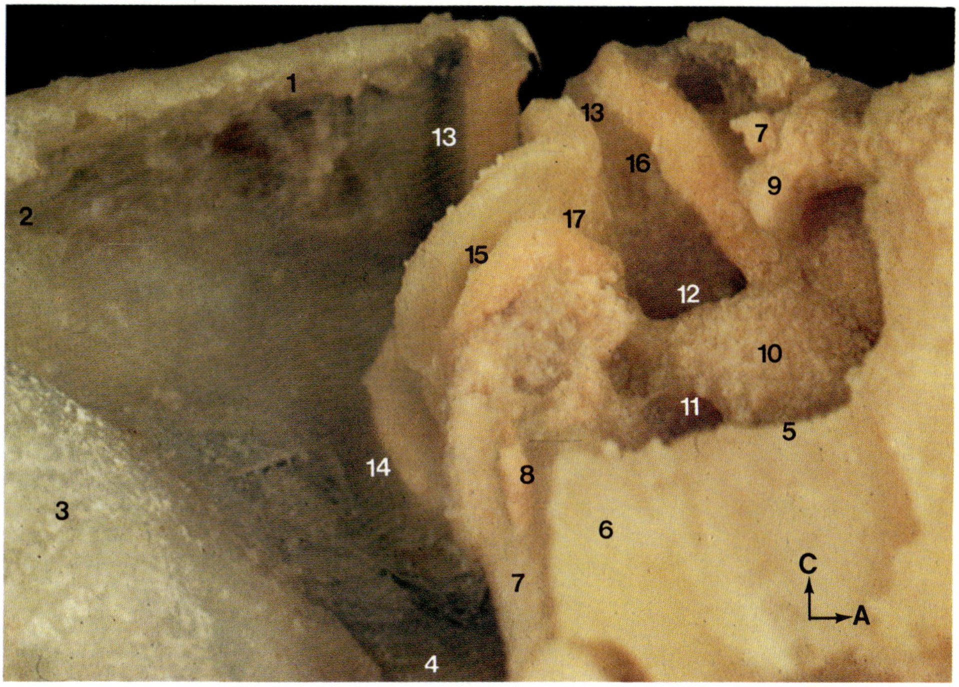

85 Infero-lateral view of the right middle ear and osseous labyrinth

1 Tegmen tympani
2 Sino-dural angle
3 Lateral sinus plate
4 Mastoid tip area
5 Groove for tympanic ring
6 Posterior wall of the external auditory canal
7 Facial nerve (cut at the oval window)
8 Chorda tympani (cut)
9 Cochleariform process
10 Promontory
11 Round window fossa
12 Oval window enlarged to show the vestibule
13 Superior semicircular canal
14 Posterior semicircular canal
15 Lateral semicircular canal
16 Ampulla of superior canal
17 Ampulla of lateral canal

86

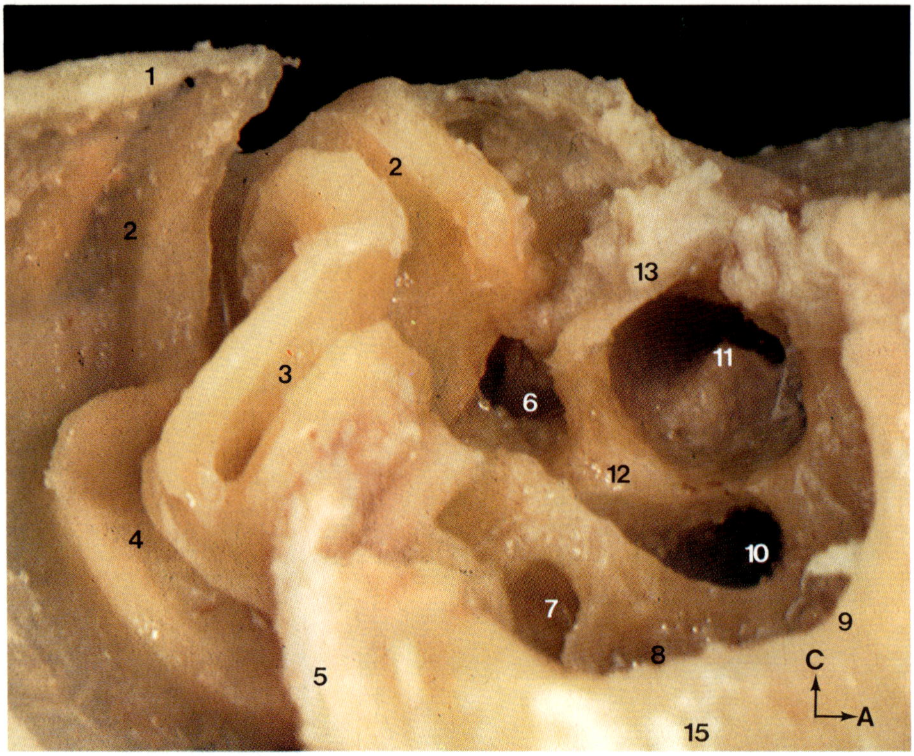

86 Lateral view of right osseous labyrinth

87

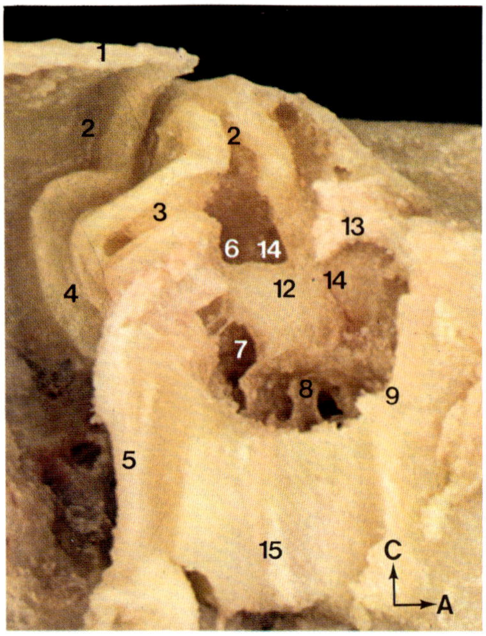

87 Lateral view of right osseous labyrinth and the internal auditory canal

1 Tegmen tympani
2 Superior semicircular canal
3 Lateral semicircular canal
4 Posterior semicircular canal
5 Facial nerve
6 Vestibule viewed through an enlarged oval window
7 Round window fossa
8 Hypotympanic cells
9 Groove for tympanic ring
10 Basal turn of the cochlea
11 Helicotrema of the cochlea
12 Residual portion of removed promontory
13 Cochleariform process
14 Internal auditory canal through the vestibule and cochlea
15 External auditory canal floor

88

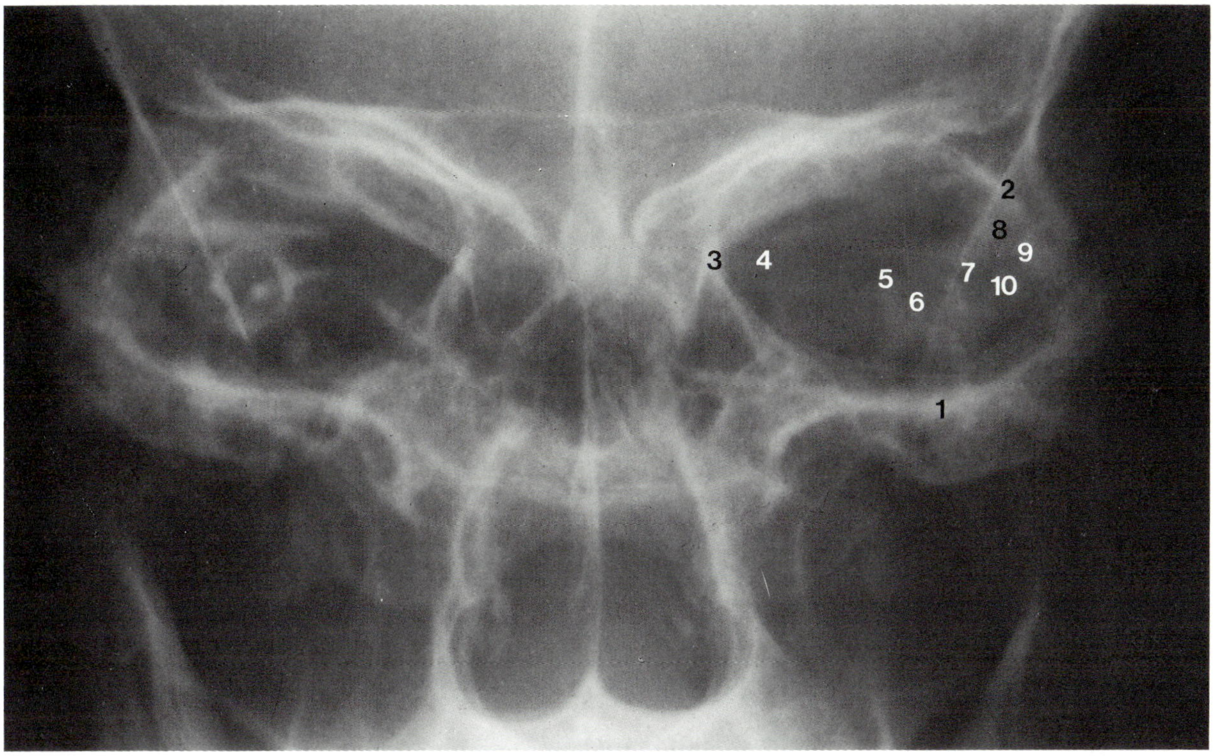

88 Postero-anterior (per-orbital) radiograph

1 Zygoma
2 Lateral orbital margin
3 Medial orbital margin
4 Internal auditory meatus
5 Internal auditory canal fundus
6 Cochlea
7 Vestibule
8 Superior semicircular canal
9 Lateral semicircular canal
10 Ossicles in middle ear

89

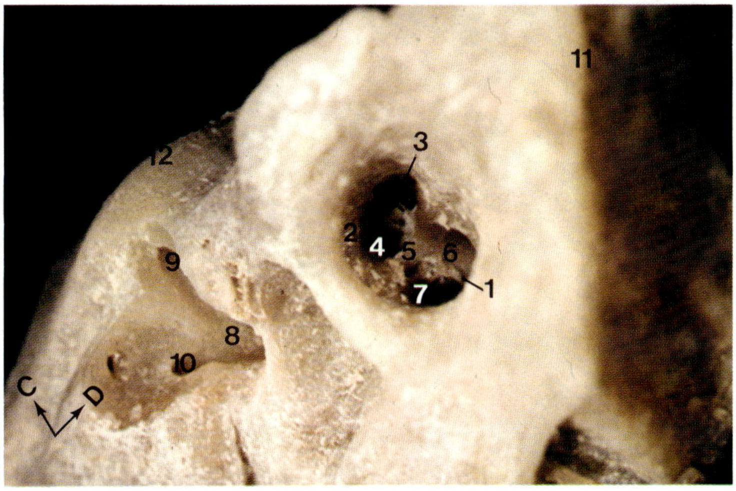

89 Left internal auditory canal fundus viewed through the meatus

1 Internal auditory meatus
2 Internal auditory canal
3 Opening of the facial canal
4 Superior vestibular area
5 Falciform crest
6 Part of the cochlear tractus spiralis
7 Inferior vestibular area
8 Crus commune
9 Superior semicircular canal
10 Posterior semicircular çanal
11 Petrous apex
12 Arcuate eminence

90

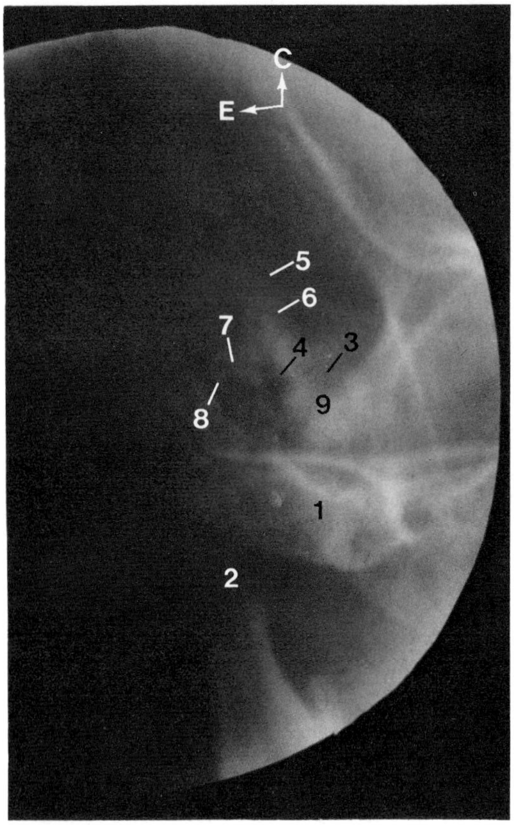

90 **Right Chaussée III radiograph**

1 Zygoma
2 Mandible
3 Internal auditory canal
4 Vestibule
5 Arcuate eminence
6 Superior semicircular canal
7 Lateral semicircular canal
8 Facial nerve canal
9 Cochlea

91

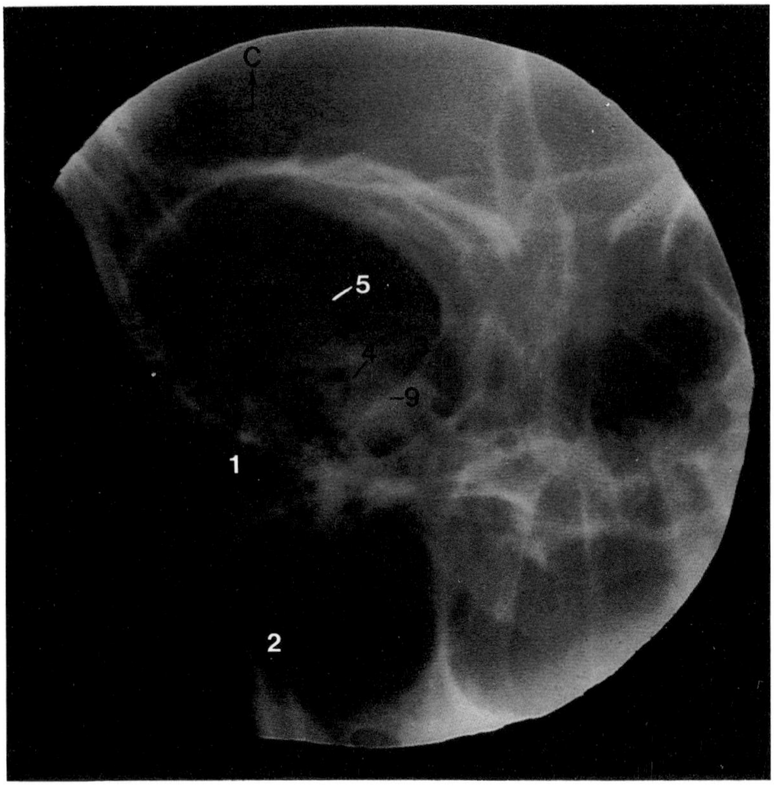

91 Right Guillen's radiograph

92

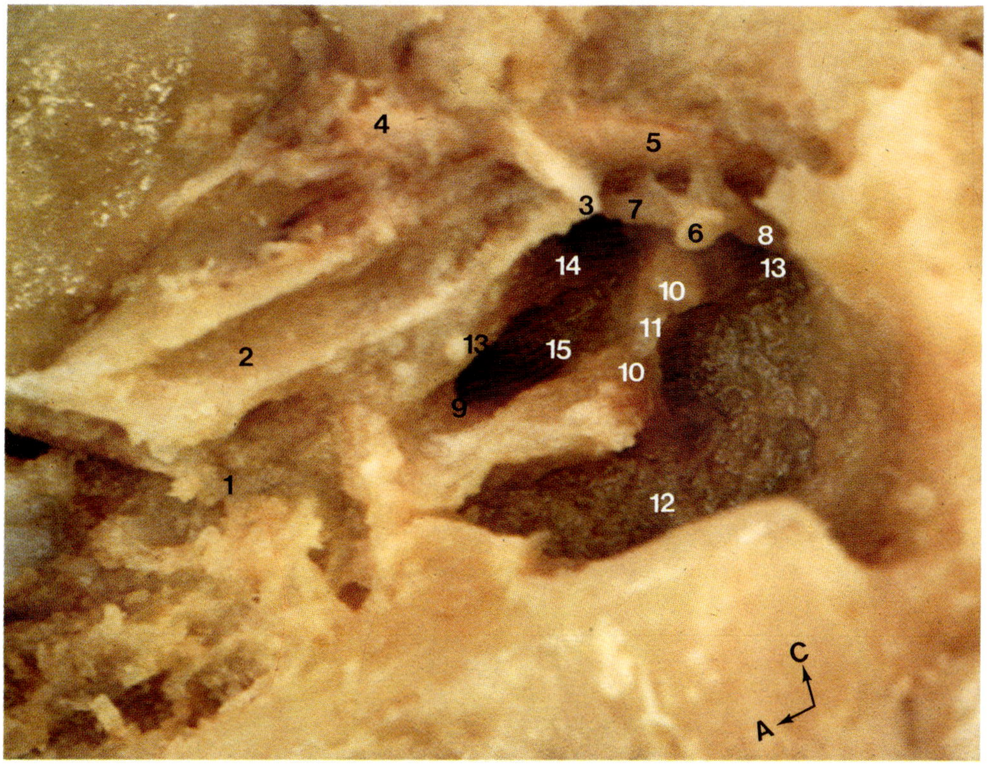

92 Lateral view of left middle ear cavity with part of the promontory excised

1 Eustachian tube opening
2 Semicanal of tensor tympani muscle
3 Cochleariform process
4 Geniculate ganglion of facial nerve
5 Facial nerve
6 Head of stapes
7 Anterior crus of stapes
8 Pyramid and stapes tendon
9 Basal turn of the cochlea
10 Edges of the round window fossa
11 Round window membrane
12 Hypotympanum
13 Osseous spiral lamina
14 Scala vestibuli
15 Scala tympani

93
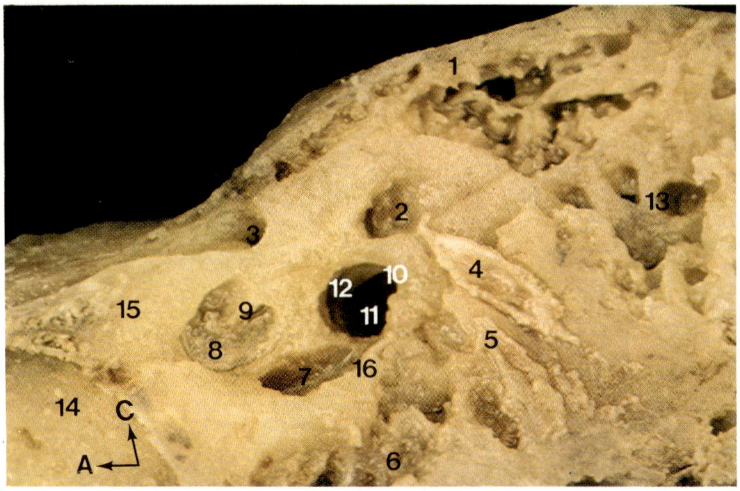

93 Lateral view of the left cochlea through the removed promontory

94
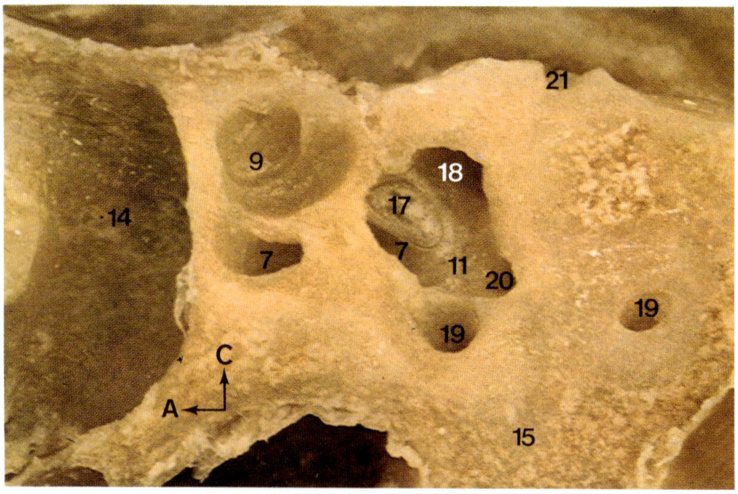

94 Lateral wall of the left osseous labyrinth viewed medially

95
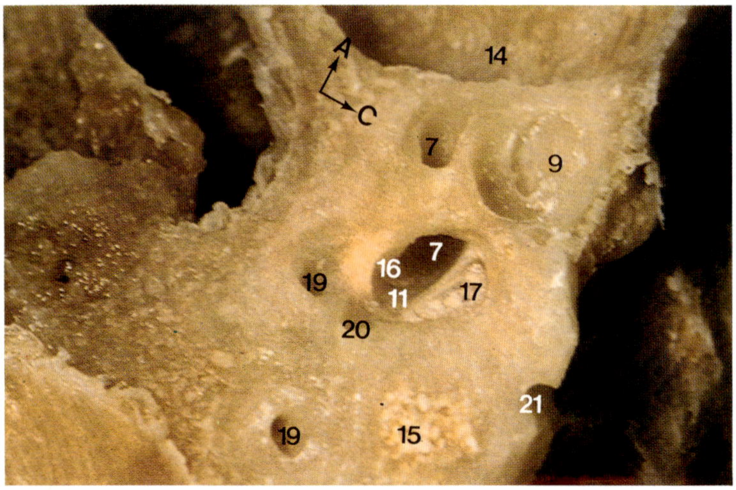

95 Lateral wall of the left osseous labyrinth viewed supero-medially

1 Tegmen of the mastoid
2 Lateral semicircular canal
3 Site of facial nerve exit from the internal auditory canal to the geniculate ganglion
4 Facial nerve sheath (vertical portion)
5 Stapedius muscle remnants
6 Hypotympanic cells
7 Basal turn of the cochlea
8 Cochlea membranes
9 Osseous spiral lamina
10 Edge of enlarged oval window
11 Vestibule
12 Saccule
13 Mastoid cells
14 Carotid canal
15 Cut surface of petrous bone
16 Round window area
17 Footplate (medial surface) of stapes
18 Area for ampullae of superior and lateral semicircular canals
19 Posterior semicircular canal
20 Lateral semicircular canal
21 Superior semicircular canal

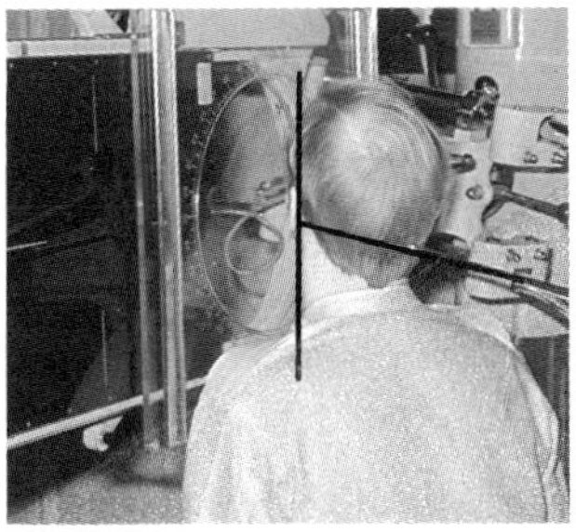

Stenver's radiographic position

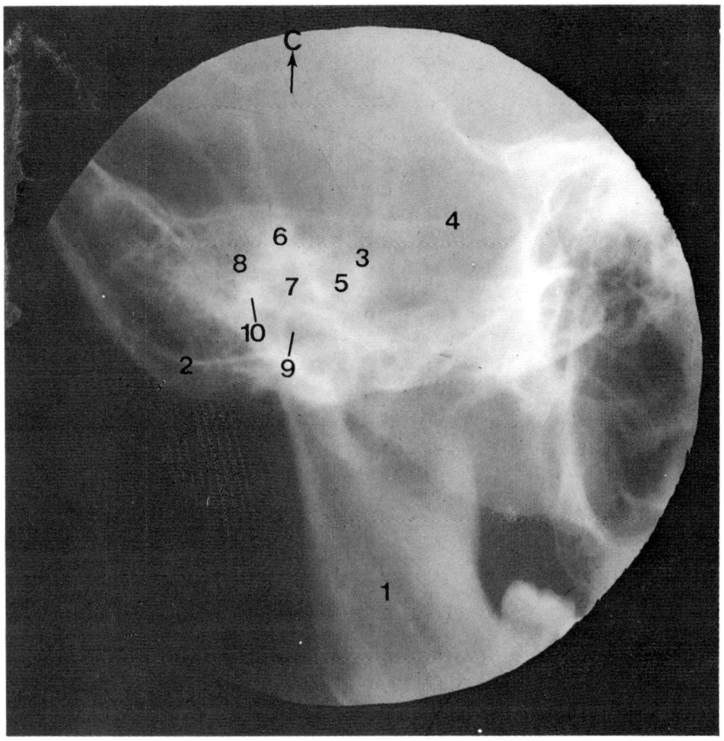

96 Stenver's radiograph

1 Mandible
2 Mastoid cells
3 Internal auditory canal
4 Petrous temporal bone (superior edge)
5 Cochlea
6 Superior semicircular canal (arcuate eminence)
7 Vestibule
8 Lateral semicircular canal
9 Middle ear cavity
10 Ossicular mass

97

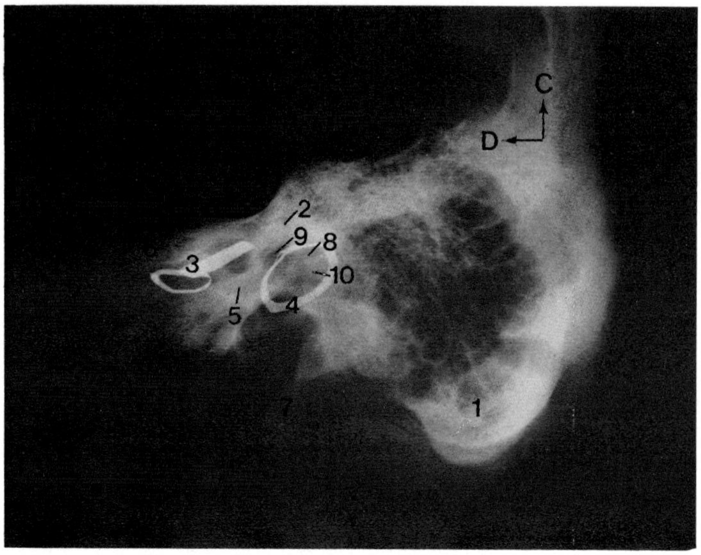

97 Stenver's radiograph of a dry bone

98

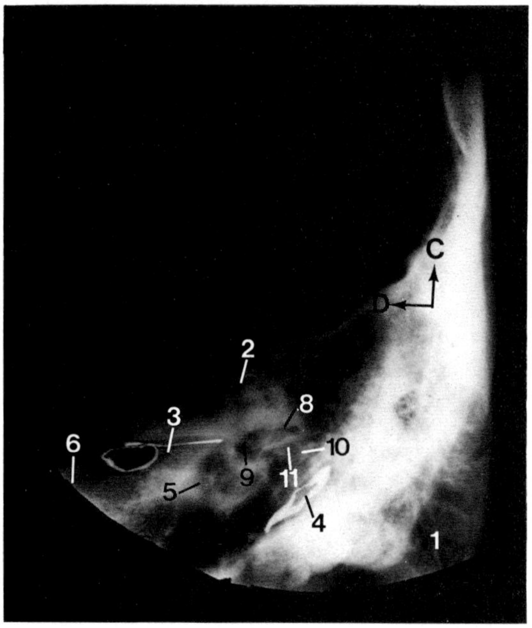

98 Postero-anterior radiograph (centred high) of a dry bone to compare with 97

1 Mastoid
2 Superior semicircular canal (arcuate eminence)
3 Internal auditory canal (with marker)
4 Tympanic ring
5 Basal turn of the cochlea
6 Petrous tip
7 Styloid process
8 Lateral semicircular canal
9 Vestibule
10 Ossicular mass
11 Facial canal

99 Left internal auditory canal and contents, with the roof removed

99

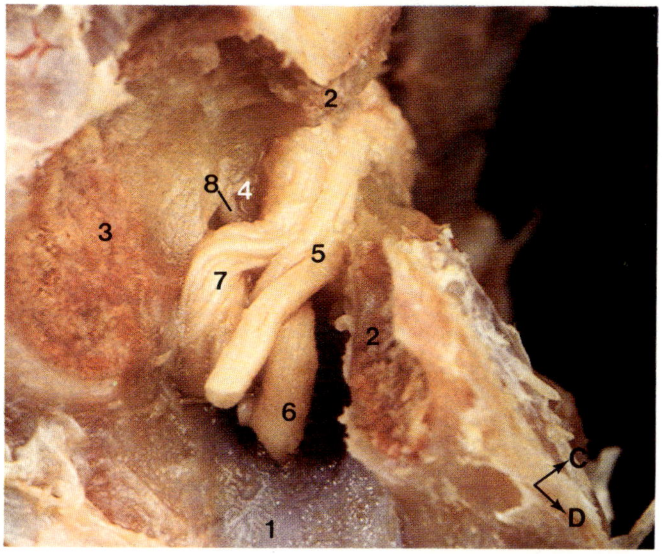

100 Canal contents separated

100

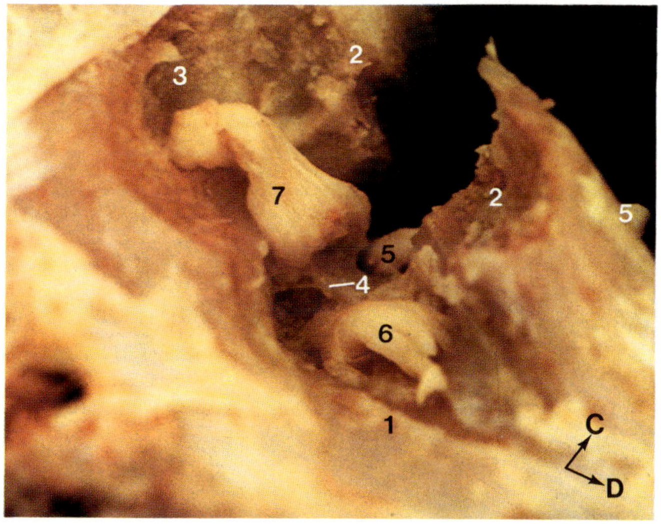

1 Internal auditory meatus
2 Edges of the canal roof (excised)
3 Enlarged canal wall (for exposure)
4 Falciform crest
5 Facial nerve (VII) with nervus intermedius
6 Cochlear (VIII) nerve
7 Vestibular (VIII) nerve
8 Nerve to the ampulla of the posterior semicircular canal

101

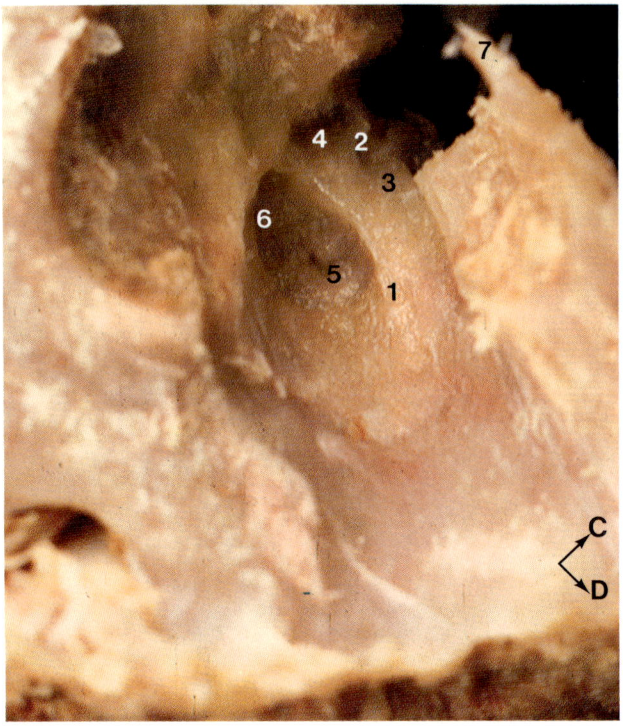

101 Left internal auditory canal fundus

1 Falciform crest (transverse crest)
2 Vertical crest
3 Facial canal
4 Area for superior vestibular nerve
5 Spiral foramen (cochlear nerve)
6 Area for inferior vestibular nerve (saccular nerve)
7 Cut edges of the canal roof
8 Facial nerve and nervus intermedius
9 Superior vestibular nerve
10 Geniculate ganglion
11 Greater superficial petrosal nerve
12 Facial nerve
13 Area of lateral semicircular canal
14 Head of malleus
15 Body of incus
16 Tensor tympani tendon
17 Chorda tympani
18 Cut edge of tegmen tympani
19 Roof of the eustachian tube
20 Incudo-stapedial joint
21 Mucosal plica

102

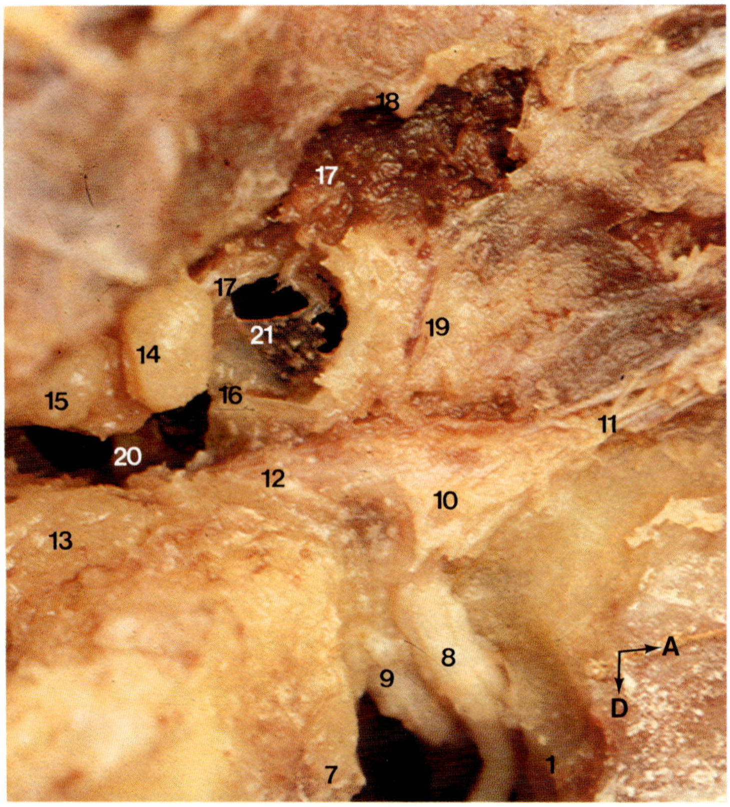

102 Left internal auditory canal fundus from above (roof removed)

103 Medial view of a left internal auditory canal with the posterior wall removed

103

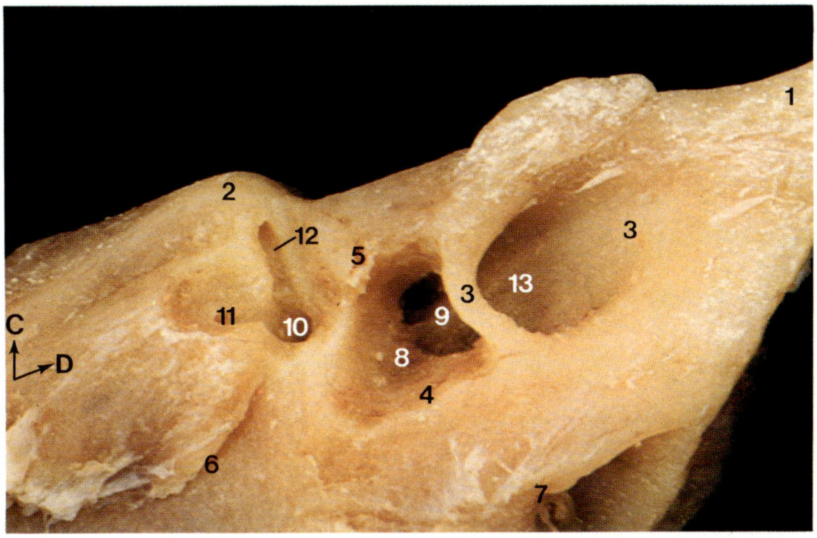

1 Petrous tip
2 Arcuate eminence
3 Internal auditory meatus
4 Cut edge of the removed canal wall
5 Subarcuate fossa (blood vessels)
6 Vestibular aqueduct (endolymphatic duct)
7 Cochlear aqueduct (cochlear canaliculus)
8 Singular foramen (nerve to the ampulla of the posterior semicircular canal)
9 Falciform crest (transverse crest)
10 Common crus
11 Posterior semicircular canal
12 Superior semicircular canal
13 Internal auditory canal
14 Vestibule
15 Lateral semicircular canal
16 Ossicles
17 Cochlea
18 Promontory

104

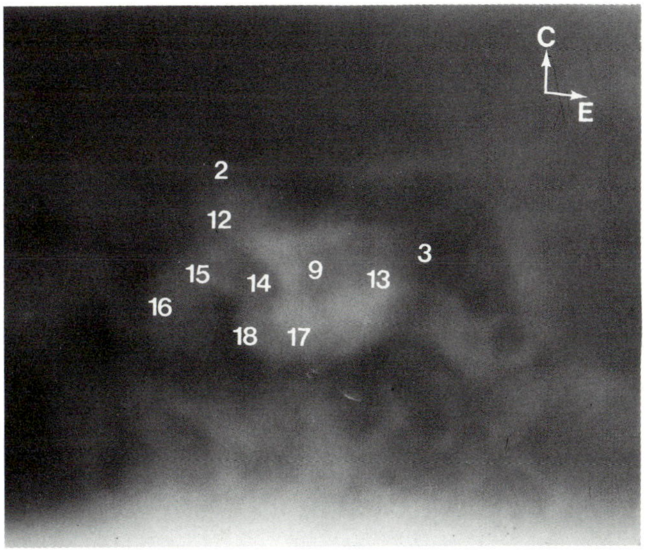

104 Tomogram (PA) of a left internal auditory canal

105

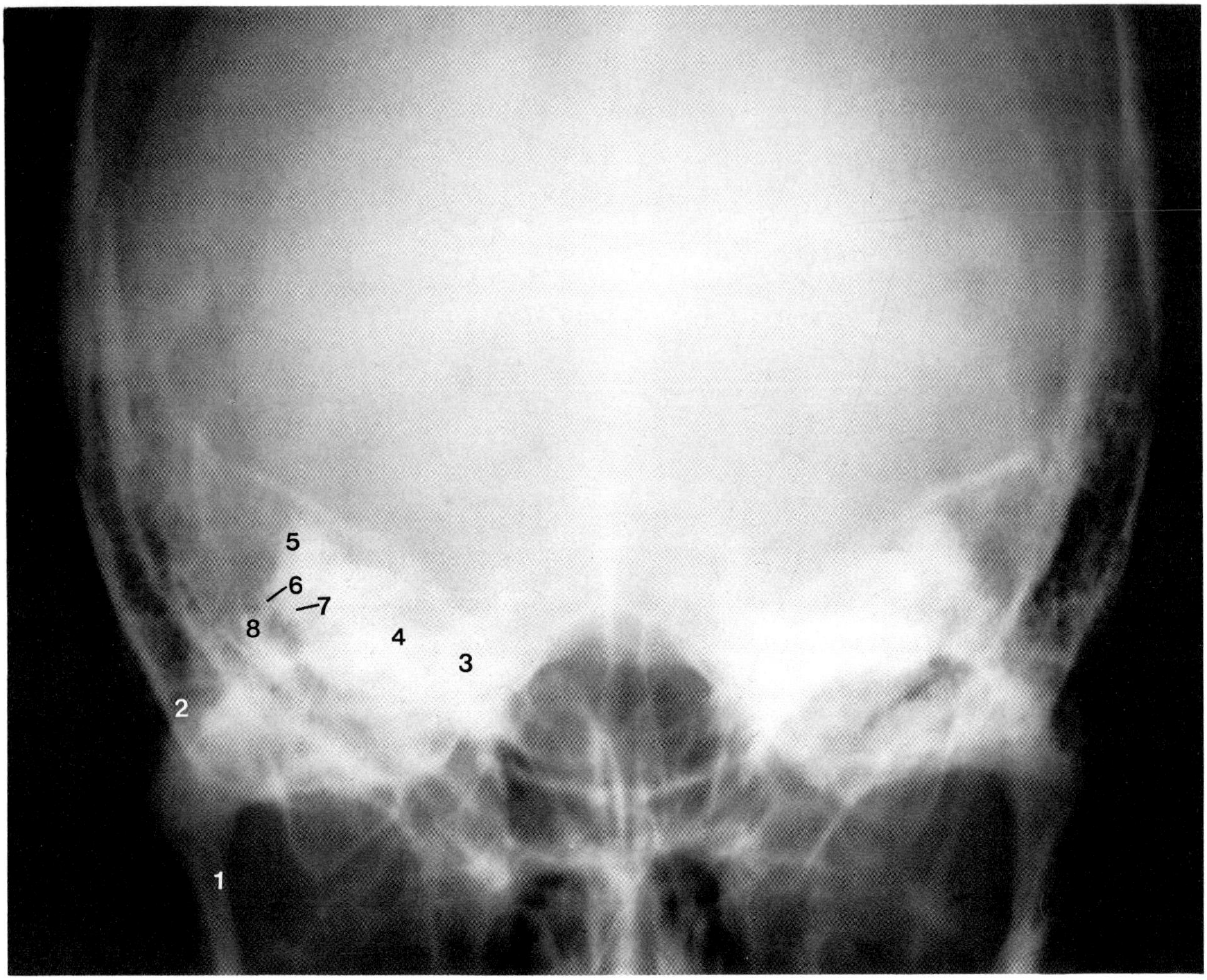

105 Towne's radiograph

106

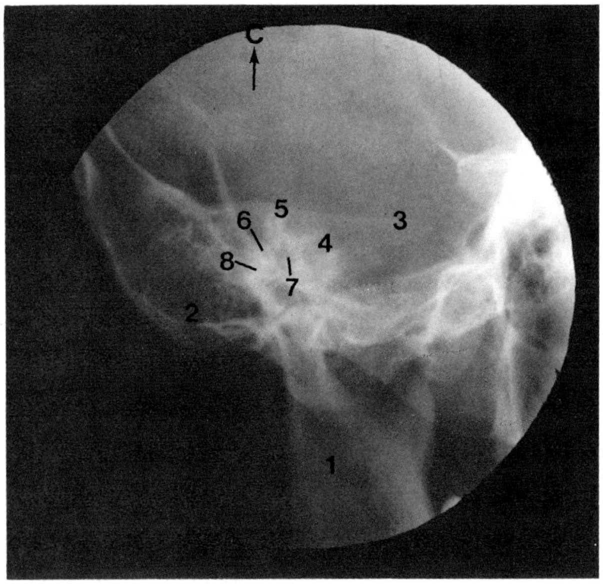

1 Mandible
2 Mastoid cells
3 Petrous bone
4 Internal auditory canal
5 Arcuate eminence and superior semicircular canal
6 Lateral semicircular canal
7 Vestibule
8 Middle ear and ossicles

106 Stenver's radiograph

107 Left mastoid cavity viewed laterally to show the endolymphatic sac

1 Lateral sinus plate
2 Mastoid tip cells
3 Lateral semicircular canal
4 Facial nerve
5 Cut edge of the posterior external auditory canal wall
6 Endolymphatic sac
7 Edge of the posterior fossa bone covering dura
8 Antrum
9 Cells in the tegmen
10 Head of stapes
11 Internal auditory canal and contents
12 Vestibular aqueduct
13 Area of common crus
14 Opening into the superior semicircular canal
15 Opening into the posterior semicircular canal
16 Subarcuate fossa with vessel remnants

107

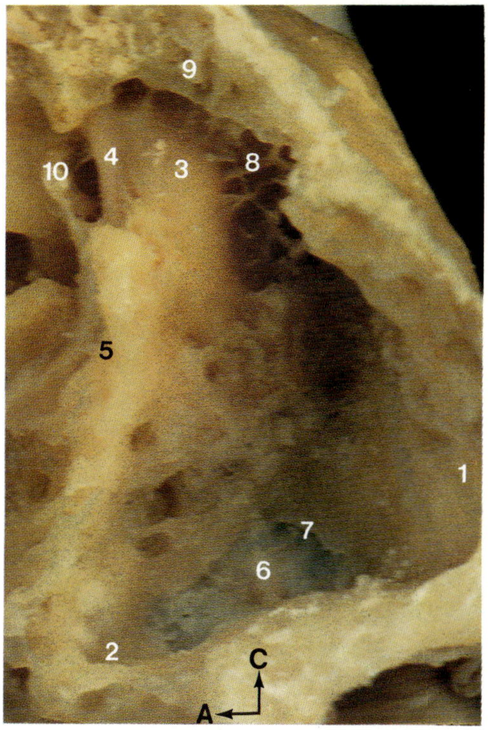

108

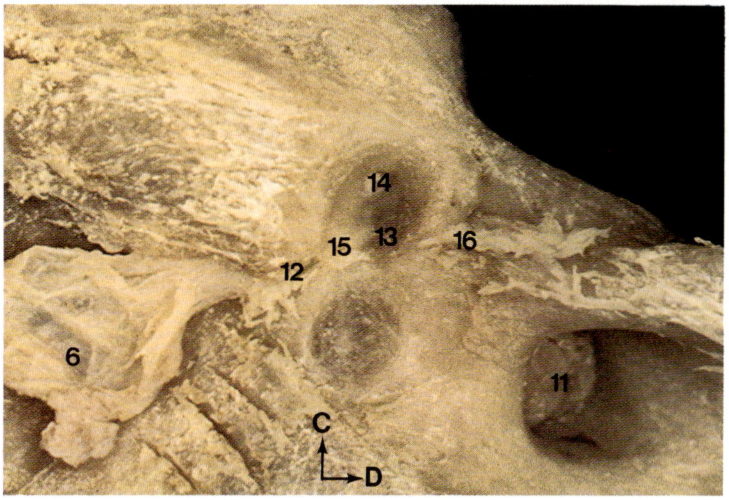

108 Posterior surface of the left temporal bone to show the endolymphatic sac

109

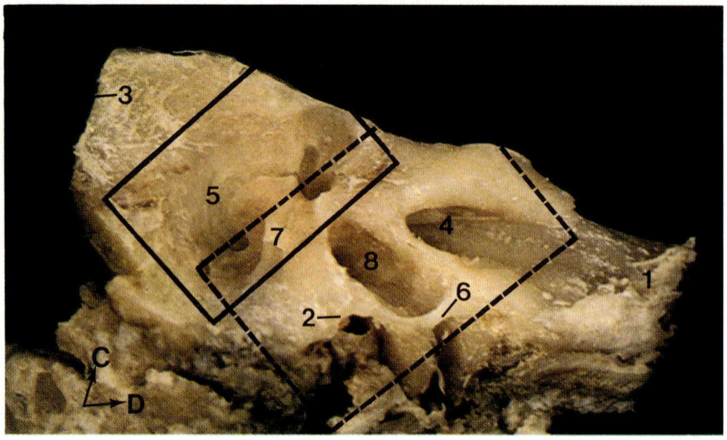

109 Posterior surface of a left temporal bone dissected to reveal vestibular and cochlear aqueducts

Note: The area within the solid line is shown in greater detail in figure **110.** The area within the broken line is shown in greater detail in figure **111.**

110

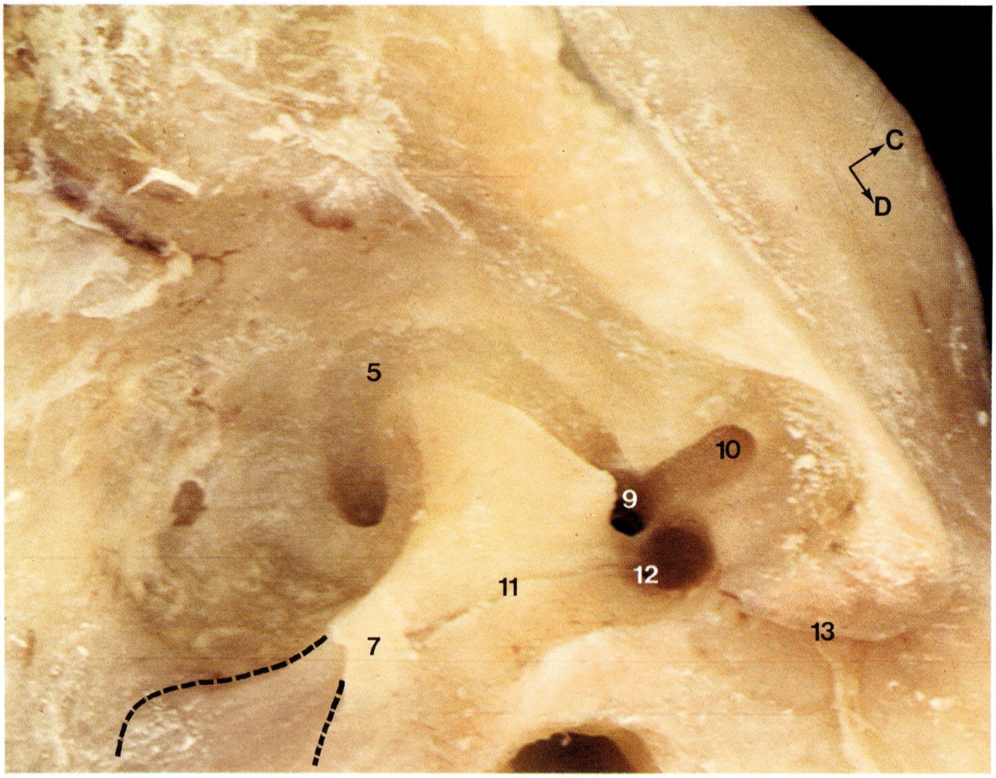

110 Close-up of 109 (fovea for endolymphatic sac shown)

1 Petrous tip (cut)
2 Jugular fossa edge
3 Squamous temporal (cut)
4 Internal auditory canal
5 Posterior semicircular canal
6 Opening for cochlear aqueduct
7 Opening for vestibular aqueduct
8 Bone removed to expose the cochlear aqueduct

111

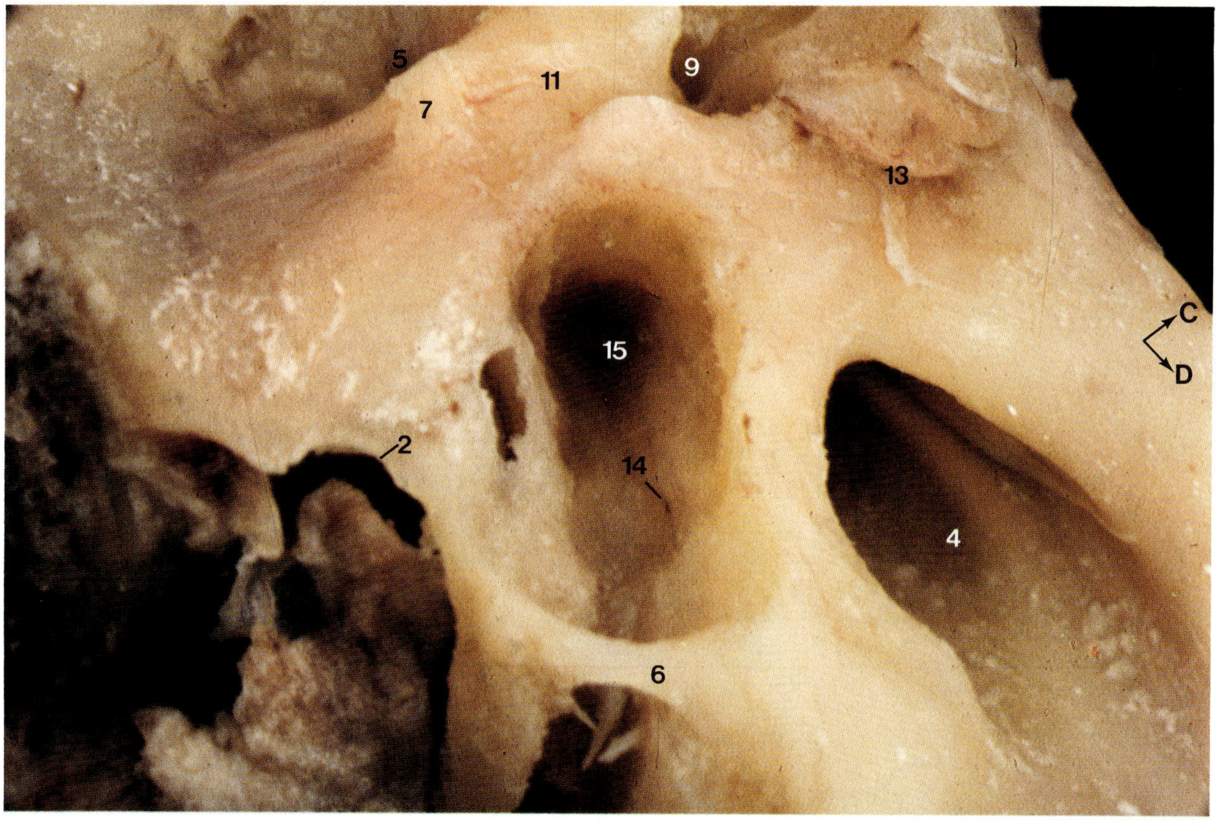

111 Close-up of 109

9 Common crus
10 Superior semicircular canal
11 Vestibular aqueduct (endolymphatic duct)
12 Opening of the aqueduct into the vestibule
13 Subarcuate fossa (blood vessels)
14 Cochlear aqueduct (cochlear canaliculus)
15 Aqueduct (not shown) opening into the basal turn of the cochlea

112

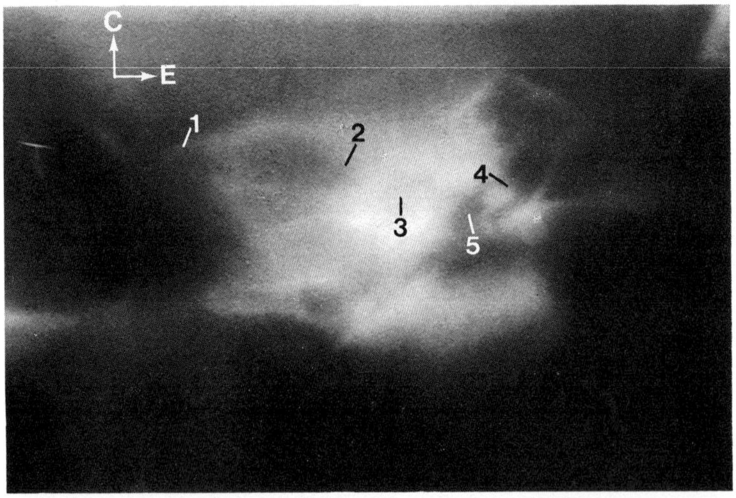

113

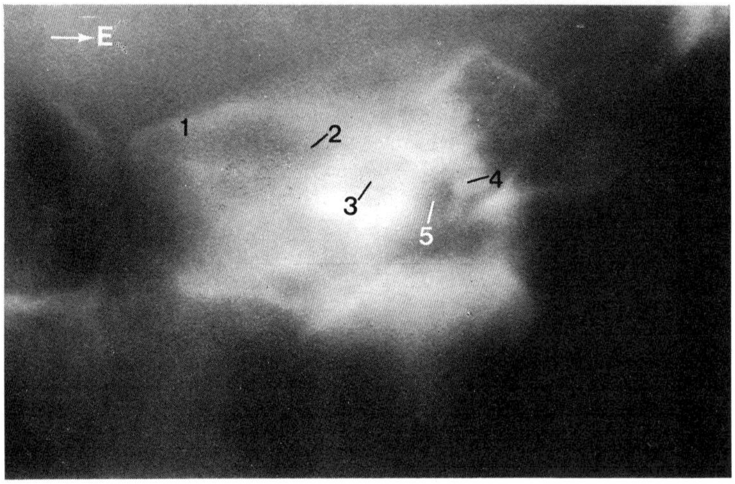

112-115 Antero-posterior tomograms of the temporal bone

1 Internal auditory meatus
2 Internal auditory canal fundus
3 Cochlea
4 Ossicles
5 Middle ear cavity
6 Lateral semicircular canal
7 Vestibule
8 Superior semicircular canal and arcuate eminence

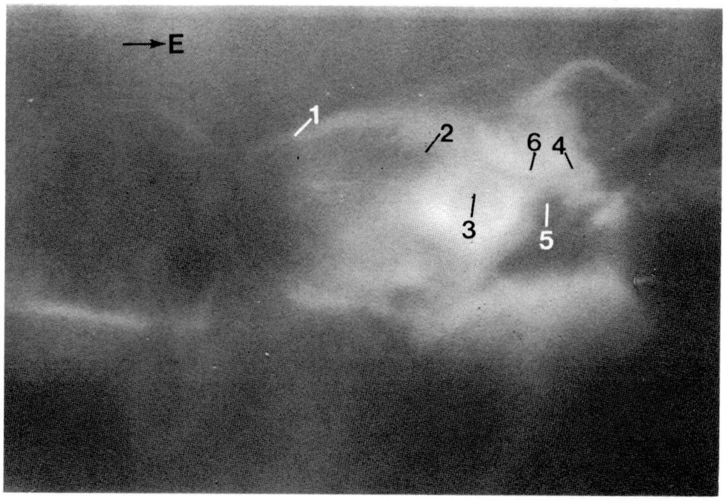

114

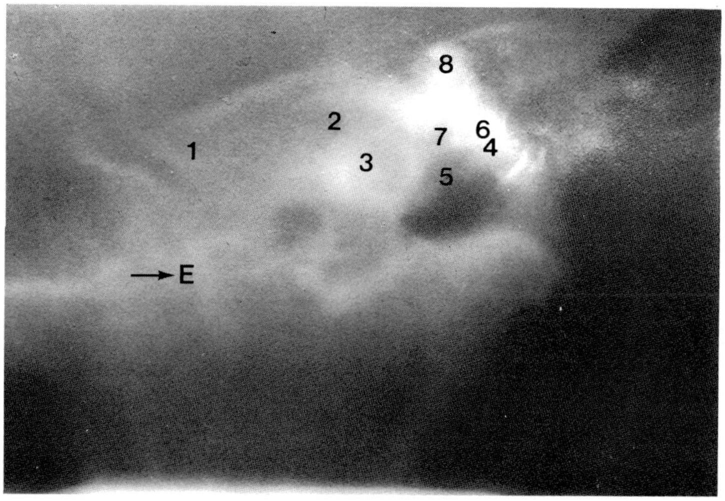

115

Index

The page numbers listed below are not the total occurrences of the item listed but only those most relevant.